Pharmacy Management & Leadership Learning Through Case Studies

Pharmacy Management & Leadership Learning Through Case Studies

Steven John Arendt,
Mike Millard, & Madeline Fry

Published by Tualatin Books, an imprint of Pacific University Press

2043 College Way
Forest Grove, Oregon 97116

© 2018 by Steven John Arendt, Mike Millard, & Madeline Fry

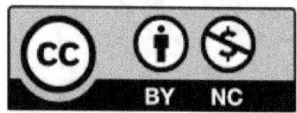

This book is distributed under the terms of a Creative Commons Attribution-NonCommercial License, which permits non-commercial use, distribution, and reproduction in any medium, provided the original author and publisher are credited.

Cover design by Alex Bell

Student Edition:

ISBN (pbk) 978-1-945398-73-5
ISBN (epub) 978-1-945398-75-9
ISBN (PDF) 978-1-945398-76-6

Instructor Edition:

ISBN (pbk) 978-1-945398-74-2
ISBN (epub) 978-1-945398-77-3
ISBN (PDF) 978-1-945398-78-0

Published in the United States of America

First Edition

Pharmacy Management & Leadership Learning Through Case Studies

Steven John Arendt,
Mike Millard, & Madeline Fry

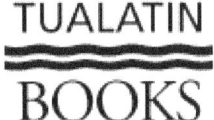

Published by Tualatin Books, an imprint of Pacific University Press

2043 College Way
Forest Grove, Oregon 97116

© 2018 by Steven John Arendt, Mike Millard, & Madeline Fry

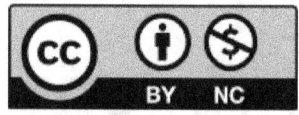

This book is distributed under the terms of a Creative Commons Attribution-NonCommercial License, which permits non-commercial use, distribution, and reproduction in any medium, provided the original author and publisher are credited.

Cover design by Alex Bell

Student Edition:

ISBN (pbk) 978-1-945398-73-5
ISBN (epub) 978-1-945398-75-9
ISBN (PDF) 978-1-945398-76-6

Instructor Edition:

ISBN (pbk) 978-1-945398-74-2
ISBN (epub) 978-1-945398-77-3
ISBN (PDF) 978-1-945398-78-0

Published in the United States of America

First Edition

Contents

Foreward xi

Introduction: How to use this Casebook xv

Chapter 1: People 3

    Subcategory: Achievement Orientation 3

    Subcategory: Professionalism 11

    Subcategory: Self-Development 21

Chapter 2: Transformation 25

    Subcategory: Achievement Orientation 25

    Subcategory: Self-Development 31

Chapter 3: Execution 39

    Subcategory: Accountability 39

    Subcategory: Change Leadership 45

    Subcategory: Organizational Awareness 49

Chapter 4: Ethics 57

    Subcategory: Accountability 57

    Subcategory: Achievement Orientation 59

    Subcategory: Change Leadership 61

    Subcategory: Professionalism 65

Acknowledgements 73

Bibliography 75

This book is dedicated to my parents William F. and Jacqueline Arendt, who ingrained into me the importance of observing and paying attention to the world and to the important people in my life.

To my children Colin Maurice and Taylor Joseph Arendt, who are two important people in my life and who continually show me that my parents were right.

To my wife Diane Arendt, without whom the spark to continue to learn, love, share, and teach would have been extinguished long ago.

Steven J. Arendt

FOREWARD

Foreward

It's been a wild ride since I graduated from pharmacy school at Creighton University in 1979. Within my first year of practice I was thrust into my first Director of Pharmacy role in a community hospital in rural Oregon. Since that fateful career development in 1980, and over the years since, I learned about and implemented many advancements that our profession had advocated for—all of which directly contributed to the health of the communities we served. I observed and supported, in my own little corner of the world, the expansion of unit-dose, sterile technique/compounding, kinetic dosing, pharmacoeconomics, improved focus on patient safety/satisfaction, and more. Our profession has truly grown, and we practitioners have gone from trustworthy drug info nerds and purveyors of drug products in the latter half of the twentieth century to coequal members of the care delivery team today. Our profession developed a unique mission among all the care delivery professions to safeguard the public and optimize clinical outcomes through the delivery of world-class pharmaceutical care. As it should be. Since 1980, I served as Director of Pharmacy in mostly acute care centers in a variety of healthcare systems and states in our nation. My professional career started in Oregon and will eventually end in Oregon when I wrap up my career in academia as an assistant professor for Social and Administrative Sciences Curricula at Pacific University School of Pharmacy in Hillsboro, Oregon.

Through the years I have served organizations as department head for pharmacies, therapy services (physical, occupational, speech, respiratory), diagnostic and interventional services, quality and patient safety and risk management departments, long-term care pharmacies, addiction and behavioral health service lines, and even a few ancillary nursing departments. As the pharmacy profession developed, I witnessed similar professional growth and evolution for every ancillary service line I led. It was highly gratifying to witness and contribute toward improved clinical outcomes for the communities we serve. I'd be among the first to admit that our work is not finished. We have much to do to catch up with the rest of the world in terms of clinical outcomes and reduction of costs. Despite the mountain of work ahead of us, we have come a long way during my tenure and I'm proud that our profession and related allied health providers are leading the charge in many respects. In the last few years, I have wondered: if I were at the beginning of my career today, where would I turn my attention to continue our profession's journey towards excellence in the delivery of care?

I started my efforts to answer this question by taking note when and where I observed our practitioners struggle and perform poorly. I observed that pharmacists and other allied professionals know how to deliver great clinical services. So, I looked for any patterns or behaviors that preoccupied pharmacists' attention from delivering care. I noticed that distractions from the delivery of care happen a lot. When "things" occur that distract pharmacists from their clinical work, they struggle at delivering care. Makes sense. Consistently throughout my career in management, distractions occurred most often with newly graduated professionals, but even highly experienced staff would succumb occasionally from non-clinical workplace challenges. The symptom I most commonly observed was a disproportionate amount of time in my office with newly licensed professionals helping them work through problems that were distinctly not clinical. I observed that clinical professionals commonly struggle with compliance to policy and guidelines, interpersonal conflict, the aftermath of miscommunications, resource allocation, cultural awareness (or the lack thereof), and similar challenges. The end result of their relative inability to efficiently dispatch these distractions led them to my office, where I helped them process the challenges through time consuming one-on-one discussions and education. In my experience, approximately 10–20% of newly licensed professionals (pharmacists, nurses, therapists, technologists, etc.) succumb to these distractions to the extent that they are temporarily disabled from performing their clinical work and delivery of care.

I circled back to my original question and deduced that if I were early in my career today, I could work at the system level as a system leader to minimize distractions, so clinicians can spend more time doing what they have been trained to do. By helping new entrants into our profession more efficiently dispatch inevitable administrative distractions, I could enable our ongoing journey towards service excellence and improved clinical outcomes at reduced cost. After the turn of the century, I spent many years working at the system level in direct support of our clinicians' success by eliminating needless or obsolete rules, improving and stabilizing workflows, and updating policy, all to support the mission of frontline caregivers. In 2015, I left care delivery and joined academia to spend the remaining years of my productive life working with pharmacy students to prepare them for real-life practice challenges—including teaching necessary leadership skills to process and move on from administrative distractions that lay in wait like traps to be sprung on the unprepared.

Once I became acclimated to academia, I came back to my personal mission to address the leadership gap I just spoke of. I looked at where leadership and non-clinical administrative skills were taught. For my school, that was Social and Administrative Sciences, affectionately referred to as "SAS." I joined the SAS team, and with my SAS faculty colleagues (affectionately referred to as the "SAS-Masters"), formed a study group to challenge and subsequently validate my observations. We committed ourselves to addressing the gap in a meaningful manner. We came up with an innovative didactic teaching assignment that we have incorporated in our SAS curriculum called "Pharmacist-in-Charge Case Studies."

Our program prepares students to skillfully face foreseeable and inevitable leadership challenges in their future practice that (as mentioned above) can easily distract young professionals from their primary mission of delivering care. Sometimes for a protracted amount of time. On rare occasions, terminally. Resulting (regrettably) in highly skilled and super-smart professionals leaving healthcare entirely. Together with my SAS-Master partners and co-authors of this book, we wrote and assigned the cases in this book as a joint project for both first-year pharmacy students (P1s), and second-year pharmacy students (P2s). Since the cases are conspicuously not clinical in nature, we deduced and subsequently proved in our application of this book that little to no clinical knowledge is needed to accomplish the assignments. Therefore, we assign cases to joint study groups of P1s and P2s and expect them to collaborate to solve their assigned case over an eight-week period.

Student feedback

During our first four semesters' worth of experience with the Casebook, we surveyed the students about their perceptions about the project. One particular question from the survey allowed us to sum up the overall student experience:

1. I feel better prepared to handle issues in operational management.

With an N of ~400 students over two academic years, 86% of students agree or strongly agree with this statement.

From the faculty's perspective, we find the project highly rewarding and fulfilling. It is our hope that you adopt this (or a similar) leadership preparedness program in your school of pharmacy. The next generation of leaders in our profession and the patients they serve will thank you!

Steven J. Arendt
Assistant Professor
Pacific University School of Pharmacy

Introduction: How to use this Casebook

Introduction: How to use this Casebook

This Casebook is a compilation of cases used in the Social Administrative Sciences classroom at Pacific University School of Pharmacy to help you (the student pharmacist) apply critical thinking, problem solving, and decision-making to common administrative-related challenges seen in pharmacies. These cases do not contain a clinical pharmacy component, in order to focus on the many other important and often overlooked administrative tasks a pharmacist is likely to encounter in their day-to-day work.

This book is similar to a clinical casebook, where it is expected that the focus is on the process of solving the case, not necessarily finding a "right" answer. The authors do not advocate for or attempt to teach specific leadership concepts in this text. It is expected that you will perform necessary research by comparing and contrasting different leadership styles or techniques and then select the technique you feel resolves the case best. Also, the authors might use unfamiliar terms in this text. That is intentional. If you encounter unfamiliar term(s) in any of the cases, look it up! The authors believe that to use this text best, you will teach yourself as much as the faculty that makes the assignments. In the process of solving a case however, it is expected that you will learn about leadership principles and law components (where applicable) along the way and that this application of the answer may enforce recall of information later when it is needed in your practice as a pharmacist. The process itself is key and should help you develop your higher-order thinking skills including analyzing, evaluating, and creating solutions.

The cases in this book provide real-world scenarios and can be applied to administrative issues that may arise in pharmacy practice. The cases have been categorized into common leadership skills, covering: achievement orientation, interpersonal understanding, professionalism, self-development, analytical thinking, accountability, change leadership, organizational awareness, and ethics. Many of these cases touch multiple categories, as is true in all real-world scenarios, but we have tried to categorize them into the area which they most address, to help you as the learner focus on the best leadership technique for "solving" the case. You as the student pharmacist are tasked with working through the scenario to develop a solution to the problem presented. As described above, there is no right or wrong answer to these cases. Therefore, it is important that you discuss this case with a practicing pharmacist in some format so that you as a student pharmacist may learn from their experiences and how they may have approached the case differently. This discussion could either take place in an organized didactic classroom experience, on advanced pharmacy practice experiences with preceptors, or with mentors. While you as the student pharmacist can't control whether these cases are used in the classroom, you can control conversations you have with preceptors and mentors. This book provides a wonderful starting point for these types of leadership and administrative discussions.

Format of Casebook

The Casebook is ordered by case number (1 through 65) and is further categorized using the above leadership categories. Again, cases will address many of these leadership categories, but the point of picking just one is to help you as the student focus your learning on one leadership category necessary for the solution of the case.

Chapter 1: People

Subcategory: Achievement Orientation

Chapter 1: People

Case #1: Bury the Clinical Hatchet

Your name is Joyce; you are a new Graduate Pharmacist working at Clinic Pharmacy. Your boss's name is Harry and he is the Pharmacist in Charge. The pharmacy is a busy ambulatory care pharmacy located adjacent to Standard Medical Center, a new hospital that specializes in hip and knee replacements in aging baby boomers. The hospital is quite busy replacing joints; about six to ten per business day. Your pharmacy is located inside the main lobby of the clinic that supports the outpatient needs of the hospital's patients as well as all the other patients that visit the clinic.

One day you are in your pharmacy and you find yourself counseling a patient (Joan) getting a 24-hour supply of cephalexin, an oral antibiotic. Joan asks you why she needs this drug. You previously had noted in her profile that she had her hip replaced three months ago. You ask her if she is going to see a dentist. She says yes. You inform her that her orthopedic surgeon (Dr. Mary Smith) likes to give antibiotics prophylactically 24 hours prior to getting any sort of invasive procedure done, including teeth cleaning, to protect Joan's steel hip from getting seeded with bacteria entering the bloodstream during the procedure. Joan asks you, "Is this a good idea?" She says she saw a TV show MD last week and he says that indiscriminate prescribing of antibiotics does bad things. You realize that this is a controversial topic, so you advise the patient to talk with her dentist or Dr. Smith.

About a week later, the chief dental officer of Standard Dental Clinic comes to you. He asks you to NOT refer patients to any of his dentists about prophylactic antibiotic use. He says that it just sets up his dentists to get into arguments with their patients about the wisdom of dental prophylaxis in post joint replacement patients. You reply that you will carefully consider his request and get back to him.

As you are pondering his request the following day, you determine that asking pharmacists to refrain from counseling patients to talk to doctors or dentists about prescription antibiotic prophylaxis is not the proper way to manage this issue. You go to your manager and discuss the issue.

After some conversation, your manager offers up the following idea. Since you have a dual degree PharmD and MHA, he suggests that you research the literature and published evidence about antibiotic prophylaxis in patients with replaced joints undergoing dental procedures and prepare a presentation to the next quarterly joint pharmacist/dentist staff meeting. It is a perfect assignment to allow you to use your leadership training and solve this tension between dentists and pharmacists once and for all. At these quarterly meetings, dentists and pharmacists usually talk about mutual problems and develop plans to resolve them. This would be a perfect topic for the next meeting. Your manager asks you to include a communication plan to dentists and orthopedic surgeons and to bring the summary of your research and communication plan to him for a private review of your work prior to presentation at quarterly meeting. You appreciate the opportunity to let your manager review and critique your work before it goes anywhere else.

You are ready, and so your manager listens intently as you summarize your research and describe a final recommendation and communication plan. What is your recommendation?

Case Question/Instructions

Please describe in your paper and presentation the summary of your research. Cite the references that support your conclusions. Include your communication and leadership plans to successfully "sell" your recommendations to dentists and orthopedic surgeons who might not warmly accept your recommendation. Basically, write your paper as if you were presenting your conclusions to your boss Harry in writing.

Case #2: Confrontation with Peer

You have just been hired as a Pharmacy Manager. This is your first job as a manager. Wow! Only one year out of school and you are already a leadership position! On the second day on the job, you meet Crystal. She is a pharmacist that reports to you. "Hi boss. My name is Crystal. Nice to meet you. Bertha is being very mean to me. Please make it stop." You ask Crystal to talk it over with Bertha and "work it out." You think the issue is over. The next Sunday evening at 9PM, Crystal calls you at home sobbing on the phone. "I can't do it all! I'm drowning in work and Bertha won't help! She won't even talk to me! She just sits over there servicing the drive-up window and won't even notice that I'm drowning and that our customers are all angry. What do I do?!" You ask Crystal to calm down and to get back to her shift and do the best she can. You ask to be transferred to Bertha. You ask Bertha what is going on. "Oh, it's okay, boss. Crystal is having a hard evening, but she won't listen to me, so I guess she knows better and has it under control." You ask Bertha if there are angry customers inside the pharmacy. "Yes, but Crystal has the main pharmacy assignment tonight. I'm sure she is dealing with it." You ask Bertha to go and help Crystal and clear the backlog. Bertha says that she has a line at the window too, but she will go help Crystal as soon as she can.

The next day when you report to work, there are three voicemails on your phone from angry customers about the horrible wait they had last night. One reports a dispensing error and said on the message that she is going to report the event to the Board of Pharmacy! You look up the prescription and discover the nature of the error. The prescription was filled in error by Crystal. You ask Crystal next time you see her how the rest of the evening went. She says that it was bad. Bertha never offered to help her, customers were very mad. "You probably have several angry messages on your voicemail waiting for you." You ask Bertha next time you see her how the rest of the evening went. "I tried to help Crystal, but she ignored me, so I went back to the window and finished my shift and went home."

Case Question/Instructions

What should you do next? So that this problem never occurs again, what would a long-term solution to this problem look like? Write your paper to solve this case, making sure you follow the directions provided by your instructor, and ensure that your paper provides all necessary information outlined in the assignment.

Case #3: Confrontation with Subordinate

You are a new Graduate Pharmacist and recently hired by a local pharmacy. This is your first job as a pharmacist. It is a small pharmacy, but very busy. There is not a lot of time for staff to socialize. Typically, you clock in and you work like a dog for a full eight hours and you clock out. Whew! It's hard work but it has its rewards. You are making a clinical difference in your patients/customers. As this is a very busy pharmacy, everyone has clearly defined responsibilities during their assigned shift. Everyone is dependent on each other to get their work done completely. If anyone fails to do something on their assignment, it is felt for the rest of the day by everyone on duty.

One day about a month ago, a very experienced Pharmacy Technician jumps down your throat for skipping a step in the inventory management process. It created problems that he had to fix, and he is very angry with you. He publicly berates you in front of everyone on duty at the time. It was a painful process, but he was right. You forgot to do that important function. You privately talk to the tech and explain how his outburst added insult to injury and you request that going forward, he discuss any work performance issues in private with you. He agrees. Yesterday he loudly and belligerently said the following in the middle of the pharmacy, "Dammit! You do this all the time! If you do this again, I'm going to get you fired!"

Chapter 1: People

Case Question/Instructions

What should you do next? So that this problem never occurs again, what would a long-term solution to this problem look like? Write your paper to solve this case, making sure you follow the directions provided by your instructor, and ensure that your paper provides all necessary information outlined in the assignment.

Case #4: Ramadan Cultural Competency: Diabetic Management

A patient comes to the counter to pick up his prescription for Metformin 1000 mg. He asks to speak to you, the pharmacist. The patient asks you if he should take the medication if he is fasting. After discussing the management of diabetes with the patient, and the need for consistent diet and exercise, the patient states: "I must fast for one month". You remember that sometime in the summer Muslims observe Ramadan. You ask the patient if he is Muslim, and he says yes, but that he does not wish that to be known. He is concerned that others will be afraid and suspicious of him.

Case Question/Instructions

What should you do next? So that this problem never occurs again, what would a long-term solution to this problem look like? Write your paper to solve this case, making sure you follow the directions provided by your instructor, and ensure that your paper provides all necessary information outlined in the assignment.

Case #5: Transgender: Which Bathroom is Acceptable?

You are Timothy, the Pharmacist in Charge and majority owner at a local pharmacy. Your pharmacy has done well in every measure that matters. You have a bustling business not only in your pharmacy, but in your affiliated Durable Medical Equipment department, Long-Term Care pharmacy, and Home Health department, which all provide a wide spectrum of services mostly to seniors trying to stay in their homes in their declining years. Even your nonmedical business (small grocery store and gas station) have done well. Your businesses not only provide valued services in your community, you are considered an upstanding business leader and have been elected as one of the county commissioners. When you are asked about your pharmacy and related businesses, you could describe them in many ways, but you are most proud of the employment you provide to members of your community. Today you are in your office processing payroll and one of your Pharmacy Technicians (Tiffany) comes to you with a complaint about fellow Pharmacy Technician Georgia. Georgia used to be known in the community as George, but after George went away to college, he came back as Georgia. Georgia meets the definition of transgender person. It is clear that Georgia identifies as female. She prefers that people use her new name and feminine pronouns (she, her, etc.) when talking with her. Georgia has some personality issues; her social skills are poor. Years ago, before she changed her gender identity, George would occasionally "act out." He would not act out in dangerous, inappropriate, or illegal ways, but in socially awkward ways that would usually end up embarrassing himself in front of others. Because of this history, which continues today, people who know Georgia would generally agree and say that she is "socially clumsy" or describe her behaviors using similar terms. She rarely socializes with coworkers and keeps to herself. Georgia is a good worker in every way that matters to you, her employer. She is good with your customers and she is a contributing member of your pharmacy and the community. Tiffany comes to you to complain about Georgia using the girls' restroom. Tiffany is uncomfortable being alone in the girls' restroom with "him/her." "I've known

George since grade school and to me he is a guy, he's got boy parts for Christ's sake!" Tiffany says, "I don't care if he wants to dress like a girl, I don't want to be alone with him in our bathroom and I certainly don't want my 17-year-old daughter [who works in the attached grocery store] to be in there with him either! He is just weird, and I worry that he may do something to me or in front of me or my daughter or someone else. We can't just let any guy in our bathroom who says he's a woman!" Tiffany finishes by saying, "Many of the other female techs feel the same way I do."

Case Question/Instructions

What should you do next? So that this problem never occurs again, what would a long-term solution to this problem look like? Write your paper to solve this case, making sure you follow the directions provided by your instructor, and ensure that your paper provides all necessary information outlined in the assignment.

Case #6: Same-Sex Marriage

You are Kelsey. You graduated from pharmacy school in 2018. It is now 2023 and you have just been promoted to Regional Manager of the Neighborhood Pharmacies chain in your state. There are about 50 Neighborhood Pharmacies in your region. Each of the Pharmacy Managers reports to you. Your job (in part) is to travel around as many of your 50 pharmacies throughout the year as you can and support the success of each store manager. Part of your job is to make sure each pharmacy runs smoothly and complies with the chain's instructions and procedures. You report to the Vice-President of Pharmacy Operations in the Neighborhood Corporation. Her name is Sandy. Sandy is the one who hired you into your new job.

Several months into your new job you find yourself at the Neighborhood pharmacy in a rural community. That pharmacy has been highly successful: meeting budget targets and enjoying low staff turnover. You are meeting with Kyle, the store manager. He also graduated from your pharmacy school in 2017. You remember working with Kyle on some leadership projects. You and Kyle refresh your acquaintance and are getting along fine. You ask him to tell you about recent events in the store (if any). Kyle tells you that he recently fired a pharmacist for insubordination. Alarm bells go off in your head: this could mean trouble if Kyle didn't do it correctly. You ask him to tell you the story behind the termination.

Bob the pharmacist, who was terminated, had recently married Steve and had come home from their honeymoon. Bob was talking to coworkers about their honeymoon and showing pictures of their great vacation scuba diving on the Great Barrier Reef off Australia. Bob was as proud of his marriage with Steve as any newly married husband. That was two months ago. At that time, Kyle says that he pulled Bob aside into his office to give him some advice. Kyle says he told Bob to be aware that they live in a very conservative community and to keep his private life private from the customers. Kyle says that his intent was to avoid creating any discomfort or acrimony between Bob and any customers, some of whom you know do not support the gay community or lifestyle. Bob said he would comply. But he didn't. Kyle explains to you that there was a second corrective action meeting with Bob after Kyle got a complaint from a Neighborhood Grocery store employee. That employee said she was offended when she heard Bob talking about his husband in the breakroom. Kyle says that he gave Bob a written warning to keep his private life private. Two weeks after that, Kyle says, he got a complaint from a pharmacy customer who learned about Bob's marriage while getting counseled for a new prescription; the customer reported it to the local newspaper. The newspaper printed a not-so-flattering or accurate description of the encounter between Bob and the customer, who told the reporter that she will never shop at Neighborhood again. The Neighborhood Grocery store manager complained to Kyle about Bob. He wanted Kyle to tell Bob to keep the facts of his personal life quiet while on the job. Kyle says he ended up giving Bob a final written warning in compliance with pharmacy policy and

Chapter 1: People

informed him that another event of disclosure about his personal life to anyone while on the job might result in termination. The next week, Kyle says that he was working in the pharmacy and overheard Bob talking to one of the technicians about going to the rodeo next weekend with his husband. The technician gave Kyle an eye-rolling glance over her shoulder during the conversation. Kyle says that he asked Bob to come into the office. Kyle says that he terminated Bob on the spot for insubordination. You review Kyle's notes about every corrective action meeting with Bob, from the initial coaching to termination. Everything seems in compliance with company policy and properly documented. As far as you can tell Kyle did everything right. Although you are nervous about what Kyle did, you do not ask for any follow-up.

The next week, while back at the home office, your boss Sandy comes in and reports that the company has had a wrongful discharge civil lawsuit filed against Neighborhood Grocer. The litigant is pharmacist Bob who claims the company is discriminating against him because he is gay and married to a man. The lawsuit goes on to say that the company has no policy against talking about spouses while on duty, and it is a violation of Bob's civil liberties to expect Bob to refrain from talking about his spouse and not prohibiting other married employees from talking about their spouses. Sandy asks you to come to a meeting in two weeks. The meeting will be with her and the company attorney hired to defend Neighborhood Grocer. Sandy asks you to come with a report on the case, outlining the details of the events leading up to the termination and your recommendation for her and the attorney about how to proceed with the lawsuit. There may be additional corporate executives present at the meeting.

Case Question/Instructions

What should you do next? So that this problem never occurs again, what would a long-term solution to this problem look like? Write your paper to solve this case, making sure you follow the directions provided by your instructor, and ensure that your paper provides all necessary information outlined in the assignment.

Case #7: Grief

You are Harry, the Director of Pharmacy in a large urban hospital. Your department is very busy; non-stop work for you and everyone in the pharmacy. Your hospital is a tertiary care center, meaning that in addition to receiving patients with complex medical conditions from other hospitals all over the state, you provide some services like a burn center, inpatient oncology services, and transplant services. Understandably the rate of poor clinical outcomes for your hospital is high (i.e. rate of patient death or disability), but that is related in part to the complexity of your patient population. In other words, your hospital treats the sickest of the sick.

Today is not a good day. You are reading adverse drug event reports. Sometimes an adverse event report is caused by a medication error, so you always take the time to review and comment on each and every report that has medications referenced or listed as a causative factor for the adverse event. The comments you enter on the reports that are medication errors include steps you and your leadership team will take to reduce the chance of recurrence of the error, like policy change, or special staff education. The report you are reading now involves the anti-cancer drug cisplatin. The report was written by the attending physician and states that (in his opinion) the dose of cisplatin was too much for the patient and that the patient was not adequately hydrated with IV fluids prior to the dose, as he had ordered. In the report, the doctor was obviously covering his rump and pointing a finger of blame at the pharmacy for forgetting to verify his order for pre-dose hydration. Immediately after the cisplatin dose, the patient went into acute renal failure and was transferred to the ICU, and two days later the patient died.

Although the doctor was clearly unhelpful by laying blame in his report, his concern over the lapse in following safety protocol for all cisplatin patients is a valid concern. Before you write anything on the report from pharmacy perspective, you need to talk to your department's Clinical Coordinator and pharmacist involved to get the "rest of the story." Your Clinical Coordinator confirms that the dose was heavy, but not obviously lethal. She confirms that the lack of pre-dose hydration contributed to ensuing acute renal failure and ultimate demise of the patient. Next you talk to Mary, the pharmacist who approved the cisplatin protocol, to get her perspective. Mary is the pharmacist who appears to have forgotten to verify the pre-dose IV hydration. You have had these kinds of conversations before, so you know how to gently break the news to Mary, so she does not feel responsible for the patient's death. You will point out that this was a very sick patient with advanced lung cancer—a metabolic wreck—prior to the cisplatin dose. Your conversation with Mary is based, in part, on professional courtesy. She needs to know what happened and be given the opportunity to talk about it, work through the grief, and use the event as a teachable moment for her practice going forward. You hope to get Mary to share her perspective on what we could learn as a department from this tragic outcome.

Pharmacist Mary takes the news badly. While this is understandable, all your tried-and-true efforts to persuade Mary to think about the event from a systems perspective did not work. She is sobbing uncontrollably in your office; nearly hysterical with grief about the patient's demise. You do your best to console her, but to little effect. Occasionally this happens, you know what to do. You personally escort Mary to Employee Assistance Program (EAP) where grief counselors are on duty 24/7 to help staff deal with issues like this. You inform Mary that she can have all the time she needs to work with the counselors from EAP and to not worry about work until she feels she is ready to come back. Mary is thankful to you for your sensitivity and support. You walk with her to EAP to begin her recovery from this tragedy. Little did you know that this would be the last time you see Mary.

Two weeks later, you get a notice from human resources that Mary quit. "On no! What a loss!" you think to yourself. You don't have permission to investigate Mary's EAP records to find out the reason for her leaving, but you can easily imagine that it is related to the death of the cancer patient. With a heavy heart, you move forward to inform your staff of Mary's decision to not return to work. Some staff have personal relationships with Mary and you can read faces just as easily as anyone else. You can see that Mary's friends on staff are crushed. While you are not at liberty to talk about what you think are the reasons behind Mary's decision, you do overhear her friends in the department talking about how they can band together to help Mary get through her grief. You smile inwardly at how genuine Mary's friends are. If Mary ever reaches out to you, you promise yourself you will do anything she needs to help her work through this and get her old job back if she wants it. You reflect how your department honestly works like a family unit during trying times like this. You are proud and deeply moved. Even though the department is hectic and at times it is hard to find the time to say hello, your staff form genuine relationships to the point of openly helping each other through difficult times like this one is for Mary.

One month later a horrible story rips through the entire hospital and your pharmacy. Mary has committed suicide! You (like everyone else) are stunned into silence. Work grinds to a halt in the pharmacy. Decentralized staff physically run to the pharmacy and burst into the department one by one. "Is it true!?" You go to the break room and turn on the TV The local news confirms it. It is true. Tears start flowing in your department. Several staff need to sit or else they will fall on the ground. The grief and devastation are palpable. Tears, sobs, hugs, and moans of grief are the only sounds you hear from your staff. Staff console each other. Some staff start talking and planning for gestures of love and support for surviving members of Mary's family. You too are grieving. Phones are ringing in the department. Some staff are answering and confirming the story to other hospital workers who knew Mary. Deeply sensitive and personal conversations begin on numerous phone extensions in the department between pharmacy and hospital staff about how Mary was a wonderful person and pharmacist.

Chapter 1: People

A couple of calls start coming in from nurses who are waiting for doses of meds to administer. Slowly you realize that patients are waiting for care. You can't just tell everyone to snap out of it and get back to work.

Case Question/Instructions

What should you do next? If this problem ever occurs again, what would a long-term process be that supports the mental health of the staff? Write your paper to solve this case, making sure you follow the directions provided by your instructor, and ensure that your paper provides all necessary information outlined in the assignment.

Case #8: Make Lemonade from Lemons

You are Selam. You just got promoted to Director of Pharmacy at Universal Medical Center, which is a small community hospital. You were hired as a staff pharmacist right after graduating from pharmacy school. According to your professional development plan, you planned to gain valuable general hospital experience for the first five years in practice before considering advancing your career into any fields of specialization. You only graduated four years ago, so your promotion to Director of Pharmacy is a bit premature and you aren't absolutely sure you want to specialize in leadership/management. However, after the previous Pharmacy Director unexpectedly retired, related to sudden declining health developments, you felt you needed to step up and assist the pharmacy and the hospital through this transition. You also felt that, with the support of the Vice-President of Patient Care Services, Janet, you could not be in a safer environment to experience a management/leadership role. You have worked indirectly with Janet over the last two years and feel a great deal of confidence that she will support you in her new role.

Janet is in charge of all the ancillary departments at Universal Medical Center. This includes the pharmacy, all the therapy departments (speech, physical, occupational, and respiratory therapy), and lab departments. At the first meeting of patient care services department heads, Janet announces a new cost-cutting plan to cover an anticipated hospital budget shortfall in the upcoming fiscal year. Janet asks each department head to come back to her next month with a plan to reduce the cost of operating each department and simultaneously maintain service levels. Ouch! In your first role in pharmacy management, you must go back to your department and cut costs, but not services. After a few days of reflection, you conclude your team is up to the task. You believe this because you have worked alongside them for four years and there were hardly any problems that popped up that the team could not solve. Yes, even in the small hospital pharmacy department, there were personalities that resisted all change, no matter what kind, but most of the staff were engaged and usually willing to try new and better ways of doing the work. You will simply tap into their collective creativity and solve this problem, no differently than you would any other problem.

Case Question/Instructions

How should you present this issue/problem to your staff to gain their support, including those personalities who resist change?

Subcategory: Professionalism

Chapter 1: People

Case #9: Policy for Tardiness

You are the manager of a pharmacy and you have a good pharmacist, Wendy, on your team who provides good pharmaceutical care in every way measurable, except for reporting to work on time. In fact, she serves as a role model for other staff in many ways. She willingly and enthusiastically takes on IPPE and APPE (Introductory and Advanced Pharmacy Practice Experience) student assignments as often as you can schedule it for her. Having said all this, she has violated the company's tardy policy and been late to work six times in the last six months. Policy says that you must apply corrective action (discipline) if six events occur during any period. Each time she was late by less than five minutes, two events by only two minutes. Staff morale has been low recently, as measured by company survey. One of the survey questions that scored particularly low was about enforcement of policies and a perception that management does not enforce policy often enough. Another question that scored low was a question about management not applying discipline to those who don't follow the department rules and perform work as expected. Yet another question that scored low was about management's ability to problem-solve issues with staff in a team-oriented manner. Your boss has brought up survey results several times recently; nothing specific mind you, just an expectation that you fix it and improve your department morale and survey scores.

It just so happens that Wendy is your secret weapon on your team to help you develop and implement a plan to improve department morale and survey scores. You personally feel a lot better having Wendy as your thought partner on this issue to improve department morale. You have great confidence that with Wendy's help, you will make measurable progress in this area. You would hate for this tardy issue to demoralize her and deflate the energy she is putting behind the effort to improve pharmacy morale. You know Wendy well enough to know that she will be upset about having corrective action applied to her and official disciplinary action in her file. She is very proud of her work and contribution to the department and her role delivering care to the community. No one has complained to you about Wendy's tardiness. You think that it is entirely possible that no one notices her track record on this issue. It is entirely possible that Wendy is present in the department several minutes before she clocks in. It may look to others that she has been on time to work and that this is really only a time-clock issue. It might be as simple as clocking in first before she takes off her coat, puts it in her locker and dons her lab coat. There are others in the department with more serious issues regarding the policy. Staff have complained to you about others showing up late. You have followed policy and applied corrective action to those staff for violation of the tardy policy.

Case Question/Instructions

What do you do about Wendy? Write your paper to solve this case, making sure you follow the directions provided by your instructor, and ensure that your paper provides all necessary information outlined in the assignment.

Case #10: Impaired on the Job

You are the manager of a pharmacy. Today one of your pharmacists reports to you that Sam, one of the technicians, just reported to work and stinks of marijuana. The pharmacist reports that she fears the customers will smell it if he carries out his duties and rings them up on the cash register. You pull Sam into your office immediately. You confirm that he does smell of marijuana and it is profound. You agree that customers within 10 feet of him will smell it. You see that his eyes are red. He is coughing, and it resembles "smoker's cough." He seems nervous talking to you about this, but otherwise he is behaving normally. In your opinion, Sam has been smoking before he reported to work. When you tell him that he smells of marijuana and ask him if he has been smoking, he says that his roommate was smoking before he left for work, but that he (Sam) did not partake. Sam says the smoke must have settled on his fleece jacket. Sam offers to go home and shower and change clothes.

Case Question/Instructions

What should you do next? So that this problem never occurs again, what would a long-term solution to this problem look like? Write your paper to solve this case, making sure you follow the directions provided by your instructor, and ensure that your paper provides all necessary information outlined in the assignment.

Case #11: I Will Co-Sign in the Morning

You are Sally, a staff pharmacist in a small community hospital. You graduated from pharmacy school three years ago. This was your first job out of school. You vividly remember from your classes how important communication and relationships with professional colleagues are (i.e. doctors, nurses, pharmacists, therapists, etc.). You spent your first years in practice developing honest and healthy relationships with several orthopedic surgeons in your hospital. They appreciate your clinical contributions about their patients the first day or two post-surgery while they are still in the hospital. The surgeons particularly appreciate your skill at pain management. In the last six months, the doctors you work closest with are becoming so comfortable with your judgment, you experience 100% acceptance of every prescribing recommendation.

Today you are having lunch with the Service Chief of the orthopedic surgeons, Dr. Miller. During lunch, he compliments your assistance with his surgeon staff specifically as it pertains to pain control for their post-op patients. Patient surveys indicate high satisfaction with pain control during hospitalization. Dr. Miller suggests that for his patients, you can modify post-op protocol pain orders without calling him at home. "Sally, just write the order, and I will co-sign it next day, I promise." Wow! What a compliment! You immediately agree! You also remember how you learned in school that it will be important that pharmacists practice at the full extent of their scope of practice in the 21st century. This is certainly that!! You can't get over how fulfilled you feel with Dr. Miller's request. You begin modifying pain orders for his post-op patients that afternoon. True to his word, he co-signs the order later that day. Over the next few months Dr. Miller and you continue with this agreement. You adjust orders and doses and drug product selection as needed and he co-signs everything you do. Everything is great. Dr. Miller's patients love their pain control, post-hospitalization satisfaction surveys are improving, particularly scores relating to the patients' perception of pain during hospitalization. In your ongoing meetings/lunch breaks with Dr. Miller, both of you feel that your agreement is contributing significantly to improving survey results. Dr. Miller makes comments about how your agreement with him should be offered to other surgeons on his team.

Time goes on: it is now six months later, and you are attending a law Continuing Education seminar furnished by state society of health system pharmacists. A member of the Board of Pharmacy is describing how he is starting to find pharmacists practicing beyond scope by writing orders without collaborative agreements in place. You suddenly realize that you and Dr. Miller do not have any written or approved agreement in place.

Case Question/Instructions

What should you do next? So that this problem never occurs again, what would a long-term solution to this problem look like? Write your paper to solve this case, making sure you follow the directions provided by your instructor, and ensure that your paper provides all necessary information outlined in the assignment.

Chapter 1: People

Case #12: Conflict in the Workplace

You are David, the Pharmacist in Charge of a pharmacy that is generally quite busy. You typically have six to ten staff members on duty any given day, about half and half pharmacists and technicians. Given that your pharmacy is usually busy, you have a "task list" printed out for each person on duty to refer to throughout the day. The staff knows that it is your expectation that they should perform the duties on their list and get it all done by the end of their shift. If there is slack time (rarely), they should help their team mates out with their lists.

Today, Kevin, one of the technicians comes in and complains about fellow technician Harry. "He never completes his work!" Kevin complains. Kevin produces a diary of events and shows it to you. "Here are the days in the last month where Harry did not complete his work, and which duties on each day one of us had to pick up and do for him. We are mad as hell and we are not going to take it anymore!" It is clear from this conversation that Kevin wants you to solve this problem and he is saying that many of the other techs feel the same way.

Case Question/Instructions

What should you do next? So that this problem never occurs again, what would a long-term solution to this problem look like? Write your paper to solve this case, making sure you follow the directions provided by your instructor, and ensure that your paper provides all necessary information outlined in the assignment.

Case #13: Informal Leader (Confrontational)

Your name is Nader and you are the Director of Pharmacy at Standard Medical Center. You have about 15 pharmacists who report to you. Your most experienced pharmacist is Biff. Biff helped train every pharmacist on your staff, including you before you were promoted to Director five years ago. Biff is also a very accomplished and experienced clinician. In fact, he is quite brilliant, clinically speaking. Biff is the "go-to guy" in the department for complex clinical issues that pop up from time to time. All the pharmacists know that Biff has seen it all before. He has enough experience to be able to figure out a logical way to handle any clinical issue that arises. He has helped every pharmacist in the department through challenging clinical issues at one point or another, and on a fairly regular basis to boot. Even the medical and nursing staffs know to go to Biff for advice and counsel when dealing with any complicated clinical issue related to pharmaceutical care. Biff enjoys this reputation and distinction in the department. In fact, he has enjoyed his "go-to guy" status for so long he has begun to behave in ways that seem to indicate that he feels entitled to certain perks, particularly regarding the work schedule. You are beginning to suspect that Biff expects all pharmacists in your department to trade a shift (or shifts) whenever he asks. It seems to you that Biff expects all pharmacists to comply with his request to show respect for his seniority and appreciation for the times he helped in the past.

Today, staff pharmacist Alisa comes to you to complain about Biff. Alisa reports what you suspected to be true all along. She says that Biff asks the other pharmacists to trade shifts on a regular basis and if any pharmacist says no, Biff reacts in passive-aggressive manner. When any pharmacist comes to Biff for guidance, if that pharmacist previously said no to Biff about a schedule change, then Biff is suddenly unhelpful. Alisa says that Biff's "unhelpfulness" usually shows up in the form of "he does not know the answer," or he suggests that the pharmacist simply go to the doctor and admit ignorance. That is what happened to Alisa today. She said no to Biff's request for schedule change last week and today when she went to Biff for help this morning, he was too "busy." That was not true, and Alisa is angry that management lets this continue. She asks you to make a policy to stop schedule changes in the department. Alisa says, "Everyone else has to turn their personal life around to fit the work schedule except Biff and this needs to stop! It's just not fair to the rest of us!"

Case Question/Instructions

What should you do next? So that this problem never occurs again, what would a long-term solution to this problem look like? Write your paper to solve this case, making sure you follow the directions provided by your instructor, and ensure that your paper provides all necessary information outlined in the assignment.

Case #14: What Did He Say?!

Your name is Sarah and you are a staff pharmacist at State Medical Center. You graduated from pharmacy school 10 years ago and have enjoyed practicing pharmacy in the inpatient setting ever since. The staff at the hospital is roughly 15 pharmacists and 15 techs, spread out over a 24/7 operation. At any given time, there are anywhere from three to no more than eight people on duty. Because all the shifts in the pharmacy rotate and all pharmacists are expected to work every shift over time, you have gotten to know everyone on your team well. You have a respectful and professional relationship with everyone in the pharmacy.

This week the pharmacist that usually works the night shift, Sam, is doing one of his required weeks on the swing shift (3PM to 11PM) with you and three techs. It's a busy night and you and Sam are fully engaged in delivering optimal pharmaceutical care for the patients of the hospital. Sam just hung up the phone with one of the floor nurses. You hear him express some frustration. "Damn! I can't believe it! The nurses Rebecca and Jim are at it again, do you know them well?" You answer yes. Sam goes on to explain, "When I work with them on the night shift, they argue with each other a lot, sometimes it's hard to work with them to time doses correctly and properly monitor drug responses when they're fighting. Do you find that to be true?" You reply, "Well, yes, but I usually can work through it and focus their attention on the proper patient-centric issues and get things done right, why do you ask?" Sam says "Well, I'm not as lucky as you, that b**** Rebecca is the problem, she is always ragging about something. Poor Jim gets caught in the line of fire. I think I am going to report her unprofessional behavior and let her boss straighten it out." Sam huffs off to the back of the pharmacy to find another dose of a drug Rebecca reported as missing.

Your brain freezes. What did he just say?! Did I hear him correctly? You glance around to see if his inappropriate comment was overheard. Zena, one of the techs on duty, is staring straight at you with her mouth open. She says nothing and quickly turns and disappears into the anteroom to gown up and make some sterile doses. You have known Sam for years and although you don't see him very often, due to his predominately night shift work schedule, you never witnessed or heard rumors that he behaves in a misogynistic manner, or in offensive ways towards others. He always seemed like a nice guy, but he clearly stepped over the line and demeaned Nurse Rebecca. You believe that Zena overheard, but you can't be sure. You wonder if this is a one-time only event that isn't worth following up. But you clearly understand that his comment was highly inappropriate.

Case Question/Instructions

What should you do next? So that this problem never occurs again, what would a long-term solution to this problem look like? Write your paper to solve this case, making sure you follow the directions provided by your instructor, and ensure that your paper provides all necessary information outlined in the assignment.

Case #15: Offensive Comment

Your name is Alyana. You are the Pharmacist in Charge at a States Medical pharmacy. You have been in this position for five years. Your pharmacy works well: low employee turnover, good staff morale. Prescription volume is growing slowly but steadily. You and your staff have worked hard to make your pharmacy successful. The majority of customer feedback is highly positive. Your pharmacy is #3 in the state for all States Medical pharmacies in terms of customer service satisfaction. The States Medical grocery store, in which your pharmacy is situated, is another story. The grocery store is long overdue for a remodel. It was the original States Medical grocery store, built 40 years ago. The store is profitable, so you are not worried that it will close in the immediate future, but you do have concern about the store's general manager Phillip, who has been in his position for 22 years. You have heard rumor from trustworthy sources that Phillip is an old-school, top-down, "my way or the highway" mannered, culturally insensitive bigot. While the sources that have shared this opinion with you are all trustworthy, you yourself have not seen this kind of behavior from Phillip. You have seen Phillip make rash decisions based on incomplete information. You have seen Phillip be rude to staff who report to him, but you have never seen him "cross the line" and demean or make any culturally insensitive comments about any group or class of people. Basically, you just try to stay out of Phillip's way. You don't really like the man, but it is not your job to like him. You are just very careful around him and deal with him only when you must.

Today you go to Phillip to talk about a leak in the bathroom in your pharmacy and while in his office his phone rings. He asks you to wait while he takes this call. One of the other store managers, Grace, is seeking Phillip's permission to offer a job to a cashier. You hear Phillip say; "Where is she from, what is her background and prior experience? What? She's a political refugee that was relocated from Syria five months ago? Is she a terrorist? Does she even speak English? No! We don't want to hire any more Syrians! Over the last year I have terminated several employees who were from Syria for incompetence. They are lazy, unreliable, and you never know when one will attack someone in public and then it will be known that my grocery store employs terrorists! No way!" Phillip slams the phone down and runs out of the office. Over his shoulder as he exits he tells you that he will come back later to talk about the leak. Off he runs to talk to Grace face to face. You are dumbfounded! That was a really offensive comment about Syrians. You sit in his office for a few moments stunned. This was definitely over the line! But no one else heard him say it. You wonder what you should do (if anything). You don't want to have a confrontation with Phillip when he comes back, so you leave his office and reflect on what you just witnessed.

Later, Phillip comes to your pharmacy to talk about the leak, and while in your office he privately apologizes to you for what you heard him say about Syrians. He admits that his comment was over the line and says that he regrets the outburst and hopes you will forgive him. You reply, "Phillip that was a very offensive comment. You don't need forgiveness from me, you need to apologize to Grace and never do anything like that again." Phillip agrees. You finish the conversation about the leak in your bathroom.

You would like to consider the issue closed based on Phillip's agreement to never do it again, but you reflect on the prior comments from trustworthy sources about Phillip's past behaviors. You find out from Grace that the applicant from Syria was not hired and Grace tells you that it was because Phillip did not approve her request to offer the job to her.

Case Question/Instructions

What should you do next? So that this problem never occurs again, what would a long-term solution to this problem look like? Write your paper to solve this case, making sure you follow the directions provided by your instructor, and ensure that your paper provides all necessary information outlined in the assignment.

Case #16: What's Wrong with the P2s?

You are Jessica, a first-year pharmacy student—a P1—at State University School of Pharmacy. You are a member of study group #5. You have just been assigned a leadership case problem that you and your study group have to solve with the help of study group #5 from the P2 class—the second-year pharmacy students. Both study groups are supposed to meet and develop a solution to the case problem. The joint study group must collaborate on the case, assign duties for research, meet to discuss learnings, write the paper and prepare a presentation slide deck that describes the plan to the entire student body. You have several months to complete this work.

You and one other member from the P1 team, Mary, have agreed to join up with two P2 students from group #5 to research leadership principles and report back to the super group on which leadership principle you recommend you apply to the case.

The two P2 student partners have not been helpful. They don't show up to meetings with you and Mary. They don't respond to emails or Google Doc updates as required. At the super group meetings, the P2 group just doesn't seem to care. It seems to you that the P1s are doing all the work. You bring it up in the super group meeting and get ignored by the P2s. The general feedback from the P2s is that they will take care of the assignment and tell the P1s what to do and when to do it. All the P1s, including you, are feeling unappreciated and anxious because the deadline is coming and the P2s haven't done squat. You complain to your P1 professor, Dr. Johns, that the P2s are not working well with the P1s on the assignment. Dr. Johns says that this is just like the real world: sometimes you get thrust onto teams you don't like, and you simply have to make it work. Dr. John's advice does not seem very helpful.

Case Question/Instructions

What should you do to align study group #5 to work as a team?

Case #17: Team Dynamics: The Case of the Resident Rebel

Your name is Malda. You have just begun your Post-Graduate Year 2 residency. You have four co-residents at your site. You form a bond and a positive working relationship with three of the four co-residents. The fourth resident, Amit, does not naturally fit in to the team dynamic. Throughout orientation he shares all the things he is working on to better himself. He does not participate during orientation meetings because he is busy working on upcoming presentations that haven't even been assigned yet! This is frustrating to you and your other co-residents, who notice that he is not trying to be an active member of the team.

The very next week you find yourself nominated as the Chief Resident. As the Chief Resident you must organize your team around various residency projects. One project of particular importance is coming up, with a residency display board to help the pharmacy team members at your residency understand what you and your co-residents are working on throughout the year. As you thought, it is easy to work with all your co-residents except Amit. Amit continues only working on his work and not contributing to the project. He has yet to contribute anything meaningful to the team projects. He will even say things like "I don't have time for that." His negative attitude is starting to affect all members of your residency team, creating low morale.

Case Question/Instructions

How will you use your understanding of team dynamics to help encourage Amit to be a productive member of your residency team?

Case #18: Bad Manager

Your name is Casey. You are a staff pharmacist at a small community hospital. You have been employed in the inpatient pharmacy for two years; it is your first job out of pharmacy school. You are well-liked by staff and your boss, Phillip, and are considered by several members of the staff as a senior pharmacist. You are attending graduate school part-time to

Chapter 1: People

earn a master's degree in health care administration and aspire to be a manager in this or another pharmacy in a few years.

Phillip seems like a nice enough boss. He has a few extra years of experience more than you. Most of the decisions he makes for the department seem to work. Not 100% of the time, but who's perfect? In the last few weeks Phillip seems entirely distracted by something in his personal life. It seems that Phillip is having an affair with some young woman despite the fact that he is married and has one preschool-aged child. You have no proof of this, but the rumored woman, Nancy, is a drug sales rep and keeps coming to the pharmacy to see Phillip, allegedly to discuss a new antipsychotic drug her company is marketing. Phillip and Nancy are going quickly into his office, closing the door and staying in there for 30–60 minutes at a time. When they emerge from the office, they look disheveled and Nancy leaves the pharmacy immediately without one word to anyone. This scenario is occurring commonly enough that the staff are beginning to talk openly about what you are privately thinking: an affair right in the pharmacy! How terribly unprofessional! Just yesterday, you witnessed one of the techs, Hillary, talking to an operating room tech about the issue in the hallway outside the pharmacy. You ask Hillary to keep the issue confidential and not gossip about it. Hillary responds, "It's not like it's a secret Casey, everyone knows!" You privately think to yourself that Hillary is right: this is no longer containable, and Phillip, the department, and subsequently our patients are going to suffer if what everyone thinks is going on, is really going on.

Case Question/Instructions

What should you do next? So that this problem (and attending distracting gossip) never occurs again, what would a long-term solution to this problem look like? Write your paper to solve this case, making sure you follow the directions provided by your instructor, and ensure that your paper provides all necessary information outlined in the assignment.

Case #19: Liar Liar!

Your name is Nicole and you have been the owner and proprietor of an independent pharmacy since you bought the pharmacy from the previous owner 10 years ago. You are very proud of your career decision to buy the pharmacy, one of the last independent pharmacies in the state. You bought the pharmacy right after you graduated from pharmacy school and you have taken a great deal of pride in keeping your pharmacy successful and positively contributing to the health and well-being of the patients and customers you serve. In fact, your pride is "contagious." Your entire staff share your pride in their contribution to the community too. You have worked hard, hiring the right people and mentoring them into being better at service. Most staff at one point or another have come to thank you for giving them a chance to work in your store.

A couple of months ago you hired Stevie. You know his family from church and you have watched Stevie grow into a nice and honest young man. He is 18 now and during your interview with him, he said that he is thinking about applying to pharmacy school in a couple of years when he is eligible. You hired Stevie as a clerk at first, and then promoted him to technician after he graduated from high school. You have taken Stevie "under your wing" to help mentor him to make the right decision about career choices. You hope he will pick pharmacy, but your wishes are secondary. You honestly just want what is right for Stevie.

It is now summertime and school is out. Stevie recently graduated high school and has been accepted to an undergraduate program. He was a hard worker during the spring and you have taken the time to help him understand the complexities of service and life in general. You are a true mentor for Stevie and you really enjoy it. It is coming up on Independence Day and Stevie has let you know he wants to take the week off and go with his friends to a cabin at the lake. Fishing, kayaking, hiking—you know, sort of like the "last hurrah" before he and his friends go their separate ways and go off to college. Try as you might, you need Stevie to work July 5th, 6th, and 7th. You break the bad news to him and he takes it like the team player you hope he becomes and says that he will work it.

On June 30th, Stevie comes to you and says that his mother Mariah needs abdominal surgery on July 2nd and that he needs to stay home the following week (July 3rd through 8th) to help her recover. You need to help Stevie do the right thing to help his family, so you figure out how to cover his shifts in your store and give him the time off. It was no small effort, but you know Mariah and the family, so you feel good about helping them get through this difficulty.

On July 6th, Mariah comes into the store to shop and you are surprised that she is recovering so quickly. You go and say hi and ask her how she is feeling. Awkward pause; "... fine, why?" is her reply. You recover quickly and say that you are simply asking, "... no reason." You ask how Stevie is doing. She replies that he is on a church retreat to upper Idaho helping plant trees on a reservation to prevent soil erosion into nearby creek.

Stevie lied to you. You ask if this retreat is sponsored by "our church." She says yes. Later that day you contact the youth pastor to find out if Stevie is really up in far northern Idaho helping plant trees. The youth pastor says that there are 10 members of his ministry doing that work but Stevie is not one of them. The pastor says that Stevie was asked to help but turned it down to go spend a few days at the lake with his friends. It looks like Stevie not only lied to you, but to his mother as well. What a disappointment! After all you have done for Stevie. Stevie is scheduled to return to work on July 8th (two days from now).

Case Question/Instructions

What should you say to Stevie? To encourage employees to never engage in this type of behavior going forward, what would a long-term solution to this problem look like? Write your paper to solve this case, making sure you follow the directions provided by your instructor, and ensure that your paper provides all necessary information outlined in the assignment.

Case #20: I Trust You, Not Them

You are Doug, a staff pharmacist working at Rex Drugs. Today one of your well-known customers presents a prescription for Vicodin #100 written for her by a Canadian doctor. She tells you that while she was in Vancouver, she broke her finger in a car door and went to a Canadian emergency room. They set her finger bone as best they could and put it in a splint. The doctor gave her a written prescription for 100 Vicodin, as well as 24 Vicodin tablets to last her until she got back home to the USA. The Canadian doctor recommended that she apply ice packs and keep the finger protected in the splint until she sees an orthopedic surgeon in the next week or so because the finger might require surgery. Your customer tells you that she did not want to fill the written prescription in Canada for three reasons:

1. She had enough tablets dispensed by the Canadian emergency room doctor to last for a few days, so she would not have to rush back to the USA.
2. She does not know, or trust, any Canadian pharmacists; she trusts you and your pharmacy. God only knows where they get Canadian Vicodin. It might have bug parts or other icky stuff in it!
3. She did not want to transport 100 Vicodin over the border into the USA for fear of being thrown in jail by some idiot customs agent under the assumption that she was trafficking controlled substances across an international border. She feared she might waste away for days or a week or more in jail before customs agents verified the prescription was legit.

You ask her a few questions about the injury and the doctor that treated her. You apply your professional judgment and feel that there was indeed a legitimate relationship between her and the Canadian doctor and that the prescription seems completely appropriate and clini-

Chapter 1: People

cally valid given her situation. You feel everything is legit except for the fact that it is from a Canadian doctor.

Case Question/Instructions

What should you do with this prescription?

Subcategory: Self-Development

Chapter 1: People

Case #21: Poor Pharmacist Practice

You are a tenured pharmacist in a drug information center. Your job is to take calls and answer questions from client pharmacists, doctors, nurses, and others about complicated pharmacy issues. The questions range from simple stability and compatibility questions, to calls from client doctors about treatment options for patients. Sometimes you are asked to perform literature searches for pharmacists wanting to advise doctors, or to help set reimbursement policy for client insurance agencies. In short, you are expected to have full command of expert pharmaceutical care. The drug information center has the following mission statement:

We are the GO-TO GUYS for our clients when they need to know the truth about pharmaceutical care!

One day, your boss informs you that you will be mentoring a new hire: a new grad pharmacist. You grit your teeth. Training new pharmacists always slows you down, cramps your style, and rubs you the wrong way. But it is part of your job, so you meet the new pharmacist John. After a few weeks of closely watching and guiding John, you have finally fulfilled your mission. Sweet success! John is working by himself now and is expected to consult with you only as needed. You are back to being fully productive and working on your own. John keeps bugging you, however. He appears not to have grasped all the guidance and wisdom you laid down over the prior weeks. Okay, not as sweet a success as you previously imagined. You can deal with this! You remind John of the process and best practices to follow when fielding calls from your clients. He keeps coming back. One day he says to you, "Sorry boss, I just keep forgetting your prior advice." Over time, he comes back to you less and less, but you observe that the advice and guidance John is providing your clients is very different to what you would do. You secretly check into his prior recommendations (all calls and information provided is documented) and learn that he is giving bad advice! He is slow, and the number of calls he takes is below what you think a new pharmacist should do. You are sadly coming to the conclusion that a job in the drug information center is not right for John.

Case Question/Instructions

What should you do? So that this problem never occurs again, what would a long-term solution to this problem look like? Write your paper to solve this case, making sure you follow the directions provided by your instructor, and ensure that your paper provides all necessary information outlined in the assignment.

Case #22: I Need Coaching Already?

You are Flora. You have just been promoted to your first manager position. You were a staff pharmacist for five years after graduating from pharmacy school, and when a management position in your inpatient pharmacy opened, you applied. Your new title is Assistant Director of Pharmacy. The pharmacy you work in is in a large urban hospital. You were selected, in part, due to your high scores in communication and teamwork skills on the test the interview team administered during the selection process. This and the fact that you have a PharmD and Leadership specialization showed the interview team that you not only have an aptitude for leadership, but the training and drive to do the work as well.

A week into your new role, you decide to "take charge" and call for a staff meeting. At the meeting, you ask the team what they would like to see changed in their pharmacy. When one of your former coworkers speaks up and suggests hiring another staff pharmacist, you shake your head. "No, no, no. Too expensive. That just isn't possible. Do any of you have ideas that won't break the bank?" Silence falls over the room like a heavy blanket. You say, "I don't understand. All you guys ever do is complain about being overworked. If you're not part of the solution, then you're part of the problem. I can't be expected to fix everything by myself. If you don't have any reasonable ideas, then we might as well finish this meeting."

Your new boss Jeremy was near an open door at the time, unbeknownst to you, and overheard your final statement. He invites you into his office for discussion. "Flora, I think you have a lot of potential. Right now, you would benefit from a leadership coach. We only offer this type of mentoring to people we believe will become good leaders in our organization."

You are floored. You just got the job and already you're being told you need to be retrained! On the other hand, Jeremy said this was an investment in your future with the hospital, so you take a deep breath and ask, "What's involved in this coaching?"

"You would have a 360-degree evaluation taken about your leadership skills. Both you and I would take this survey, plus colleagues and other managers inside and outside the pharmacy that you select. It's a survey that assesses emotional intelligence, or EI. We know managers who have strong emotional intelligence skills outperform those who don't. We don't do this just to be nice: it's good business. EI encompasses self-awareness, self-regulation, self-motivation, social awareness, and social skills, and within each of these areas, specific skill sets."

You agree to participate in the 360-degree evaluation and EI coaching. When you read the results of the evaluation, the following scores upset you:
- Adaptable/Flexible: 60% (normal range 64–80%)
- Communication: 62% (normal range 66–83%)
- Emotional Self-Awareness: 70% (normal range 61–81%)
- Empathy: 59% (normal range 61–80%)

The feedback on empathy is the most distressing. You always assumed you excelled in that competency. Don't you always ask your people for input? Aren't you always available? Or so you thought: clearly, others do not see you the way you see yourself.

At your first one-on-one session, your coach asks what you want to get out of the experience. You answer, "I want to be a better listener in order to improve my ability to show empathy."

For the first month, the coach has you focus on your listening skills. You have one-on-one meetings with every member of your staff and ask what you can do to make their jobs better. You keep a notebook of observations of when listening experiences go well and when they go poorly. After a two-week period, you review your notes and conclude that your best listening and best outcomes occurred when:
- you are prepared with script, notes, data, lists, and plans;
- you trust the other person; and,
- you are calm and relaxed.

You also find your worst listening and worst outcomes occurred when:
- you feel under attack or sandbagged;
- you are told your facts/perceptions are not real; and,
- old history is dredged up, not relevant to the situation at hand.

Armed with this new perspective about your leadership abilities, you are eager to try another staff meeting and solicit input from your team about changes they would like. Sure enough, when you ask the question, the same coworker asks for more staff pharmacists, just like last time. Instead of responding the same way as last time, you respond differently...

Case Question/Instructions

How should you respond to the request to add more staff?

Case #23: Behavioral Interviewing

Your name is Summer, and you are a newly hired manager in a hospital pharmacy. You have been on the job for three months. Your boss, Lars, the hospital's Chief Nursing Officer, is a surly old codger but you have had no embarrassing moments or arguments with him and he seems responsive enough to your requests for information. You are kind of intimidated

Chapter 1: People

by him, but you are working on getting over that, so you can concentrate on being a great manager and leader for your pharmacy department.

You have just been informed that your request to hire two Pharmacy Technicians has been approved. These are your first hires since you started the job, so you want to show your appreciation to Lars by hiring two top-notch techs. It is a good way for you to collaborate with your new staff too. So, you find yourself all jazzed up and ready to go!

Despite your best efforts, and that of your staff, to select good techs, your two new hires fizzle out and are terminated within three months of hire, during their probationary period. When you reflect on what went wrong, you conclude that you and your team really didn't know what you were getting when you hired them. The techs were not articulate, didn't care, got into arguments with your staff and customers, and did shoddy work. You are glad they are gone, but now you must go to Lars and ask for two replacement positions.

In your meeting with Lars, you explain what happened and your conclusion that the techs did not represent themselves accurately during interview. Lars asks you if you know about behavioral interviewing. You search your memories and must confess that you don't remember at this moment. Lars asks you to develop some behavioral interview questions that reveal the deficiencies you found in your former techs, so he can be convinced that the next techs you hire won't have the same bad habits. He goes onto say that until you demonstrate to him that you can ask appropriate behavioral interview questions that can allow you to detect personality deficiencies, he will not approve any replacement positions for your department.

The decision is painful but seems fair. At least he gave you a way forward out of this mess and there is a chance that you can get two replacement positions approved. You do some research into behavioral interviewing and realize that you know all about it from pharmacy school. You quickly begin work with some of your staff to develop some appropriate interview questions that will allow you and your team to detect personality flaws in applicants before they are hired.

Case Question/Instructions

Your paper (and subsequent presentation) need to explain the differences between behavioral interview questions and traditional interview questions and cite some references that support your definition and appropriate application of behavioral questioning in a job interview setting. Your paper needs to explain what questions are illegal, so Lars can see that you understand and can protect the company by not asking questions that are not allowed by law. Your paper needs to provide at least two behavioral interview questions that can allow you and your team to detect any personality deficiencies in the following categories:

- *Communication skills*
- *Commitment to work and company*
- *Quality of work*
- *Problem solving*
- *Teamwork*

Chapter 2: Transformation

Subcategory: Achievement Orientation

Chapter 2: Transformation

Case #24: CPR Policy

You are a staff pharmacist at a large community chain pharmacy. Your boss (Mariah) is the Vice-President of Pharmacy Operations for the chain of pharmacies where you work. Mariah has several regional pharmacy managers that work for her. Over the years you have worked for the company, you have observed that Regional Managers tend to come and go. You seek to apply for the next vacancy that occurs. Accordingly, you have shared your personal professional development plan with your boss and Mariah and you have specifically informed her that you will apply when the next vacancy for Regional Manager occurs. Mariah acknowledged your professional goal and informs you that she will keep your interest in mind.

Several months later Mariah is visiting your store and asks you to join her in your manager's office. She tells you that she remembers your interest in becoming a Regional Manager and asks if you would be willing to take on a project that she would normally give to one of her Regional Managers. She says it will give you a taste of the kind of work a Regional Manager does. You quickly accept her offer and ask her how you can help! Mariah tells you of a complaint from a patient's family at another store. She says that family is threatening to sue because they are so upset. Mariah says that the company needs a policy to help demonstrate to the family that the company is taking the event very seriously and wants to improve. She asks if you are willing to write that policy. You say "Of course!" You ask Mariah to provide you with some back ground.

Two months ago, a long-time patient in another pharmacy collapsed from a heart attack while in the pharmacy. The pharmacist on duty, Joseph, called 911 and immediately carried out CPR on the patient until the paramedics arrived. The patient did not survive the event and died en route to the hospital. Later that day, Joseph was attempting to comfort grieving family through their loss and somehow it was revealed to the family that our company does not provide CPR training to our pharmacists and that Joseph's CPR certification, which he earned while attending State University School of Pharmacy, expired two years ago. The brother of the patient got mad and is threatening to sue us for this gross negligence. Mariah asks that, while you are drafting our company policy about CPR, you research whatever law might exist to protect the company from such a lawsuit and make sure the draft policy complies with all state rules pertaining to administering CPR in public. She asks you to provide some basic analysis of how much the implementation of your draft policy will cost if the company adopts your draft policy unchanged.

Case Question/Instructions

When you write your paper to solve this case, include a draft policy with ballpark cost estimates. No special format is required. You can copy a policy format from IPPE (Introductory Pharmacy Practice Experience) rotation sites, or make one up on your own.

Case #25: Computerized Physician Order Entry

You are the Director of Pharmacy at State General Hospital. You are in charge of the inpatient pharmacy. You were hired into this position 6 months ago, and only 10 months after graduation from State University School of Pharmacy. You vividly remember your medication safety and how easy it is to hurt or even kill patients through prescribing errors in hospitals. That is why you are extremely happy to learn that your hospital has just entered into a contract with a company to upgrade your hospital information system, which will require doctors to enter orders directly into the computer, thus eliminating the chance your staff will make an error reading sloppy handwritten orders on paper.

Doctors, nurses, and your staff have all received training. Everything is ready to "go live". The entire hospital is buzzing with excitement and apprehension. The day comes and nothing much happens. It was a slow day for your pharmacists. Hospital census was normal, but the number of orders was really low. You go to the hospital leadership debriefing at the end of the first day on the new system and are shocked to hear the doctors are very upset with the new system. It takes them forever to enter new orders and wade through all the alerts the system forces them to click through. They need to hire four more doctors just to keep up! Since the doctors are employed by the hospital, administrators immediately veto that idea. Then the doctors state that they want to go back to handwriting orders for the next six months while all the bugs are worked out and have the pharmacists enter the orders. Either this or they will start transferring their patients to the other hospital across town! Every department head present at the meeting, including your boss, turns to you. Can you do this?

Case Question/Instructions

How do you respond? Is there a "teachable" moment for your boss, the doctors, and the entire management team of the hospital? What is that? How and when should you communicate that?

Case #26: United We Stand

You are Boupha, the newly hired Director of Operations at State Care Rx, a long-term care (LTC) pharmacy that supports members in LTC facilities (nursing homes) and hospice care facilities. You were hired to help the pharmacy make it through a recent serious spike in growth. The marketing department at State Care Rx recently signed contracts with 10 LTC facilities. These 10 new nursing homes represent a 100% growth in LTC beds served by State Care Rx. An astonishing growth spurt, which some executives in the company fear can't be done safely. So you were recruited: you have many years of experience successfully leading large LTC pharmacies through change. Upon hire, the first thing you did was convince the Board that you needed some Operational Coordinators. One for Quality and Safety, and another for the Clinical and Practice activities of all the pharmacists on staff. It was an easy sell, since several members of the Board shared executive concerns about the safety and wisdom of such rapid growth at State Care Rx. You quickly hire your two new coordinators, Truc and Tom. Since these were new positions in the company, both Truc and Tom knew that they would have the freedom (and the burden) of making their contributions valuable for the company. In other words, there was no history or track record for either position that they could use to help guide their work or measure their success. You took the time needed to explain how you thought Tom and Truc should collaborate to ensure safety and quality of the services State Care Rx provided all their patients.

Several months into their new roles, you meet regularly with Truc and Tom together and with each of them individually. It is becoming apparent that the two Operational Coordinators are having difficulty knowing where one person's responsibility ends and the other's begins. Time and time again, one coordinator tells you that the other coordinator "needs to handle it" or to "back off and let me handle it." It is clear to you now that your initial effort to explain the respective roles of the two coordinators was insufficient. This discovery is not a failure on anyone's part, but it will become a large problem if not addressed quickly. You remember that these were two newly created positions and so "wrinkles" like this should be expected.

Case Question/Instructions

How should you proceed with resolving the conflict that exists between the two in an empowering manner that does not disenfranchise ether coordinator?

Case #27: Avalanche

You are Linda, a recent graduate from a school of pharmacy. Right out of school you landed a job as a Director of Pharmacy. The hospital is small and the staff is small, but you are quite pleased with your new job. Not only is it consistent with your career development plan, you

Chapter 2: Transformation

look forward to practicing the leadership skills you learned in school. After the first few months on the job, you are happy with the outcomes thus far. Your small staff seems to get along with you; the nurses and doctors have developed a genuine relationship with you, and you feel that your patients are getting good pharmaceutical care. You start to expand your experiences by volunteering in statewide pharmacy professional organizations (more than one) and local civic leadership activities. All these decisions are part of your career development plan. On top of that, you've found a boyfriend and it looks like he might end up being "the one!"

Time goes on and your responsibilities at work grow. Your responsibilities in local and state professional organizations grow too. Your boyfriend is now your husband, and you have bought a new home and can't wait to start a family. There are many competing priorities in your professional and personal life. Some priorities are more enjoyable than others. Your staff at work have begun to make comments about you not being as "present" or engaged as you were when you first started the job. Nurses and doctors have been heard commenting about being disappointed in your work because you're taking too many shortcuts or not thinking through all available options before making decisions. Other aspects of your life are going smoothly, like the home improvement projects with your husband and in your neighborhood. You enjoy the time you spend at home and with friends and neighbors, and you are finding yourself spending more time on these enjoyable activities. It is beginning to affect the quality of your work as you spend less and less time and energy with pharmacy and hospital-related issues.

Today you are meeting with your boss, the Chief Nursing Officer Cindy. Cindy begins to list the deficiencies she is noticing with your work. Poor selection of replacement staff, higher turnover among your staff, higher rate of medication errors originating in the pharmacy, more frequent patient complaints about the service from pharmacy, slower responsiveness from you when presented with problems that need the pharmacy's perspective, lower staff morale according to a hospital-wide employee survey, and more. Cindy points out that you have a 24/7 responsibility to the hospital and your department, and you can't just clock out at the end of the day or week and trust that things will go well in your absence. Cindy summarizes what she thinks is going on: "Linda, I think you have too much going on in your life and your department is suffering. I think you might want to dial it back a little." You are upset. You can't disagree with the long list of issues Cindy just presented. You admit to yourself that you have been experiencing more and more frequent feelings of being overwhelmed with all the work you must do, and too often you are failing to meet others' expectations. The idea of just dropping things off your plate to create more time for the more important priorities in your life seems like a step backward. Cindy gives you a month to come back with a plan to address declining work quality.

Case Question/Instructions

Please develop a plan that addresses Cindy's concerns.

Case #28: Total Parenteral Nutrition Upgrades

You are Myrsady, an experienced pharmacist at one of the outlying health system hospital pharmacies. Since being hired five years ago, you have developed an interest in total parenteral nutrition (TPN) in adults and typically spend anywhere from 30 to 60 minutes each day working with dieticians and doctors to calculate calories, electrolytes, and other trace ingredients needed by each patient receiving TPN at your hospital. The patients don't do TPN every day, and are usually discharged or transferred after 1–3 days on TPN, so the pharmacy, nurses, and doctors and dieticians appreciate your experienced help working with the interdisciplinary team to appropriately determine each patient's nutritional needs.

The Chief Pharmacy Officer (CPO) for inpatient pharmacies in the health system home office is concerned that too many outlying hospitals are spending too many resources on management of TPN when there is little evidence that anything is needed beyond a standardized formula of amino acids, fats, and dextrose. The pharmacy home office has just invested in a computer program that allows doctors or even technicians to enter certain patient parameters and conditions and receive a basic, fairly standardized TPN formula for the pharmacy to compound. It does not try to address every nutritional aspect of the patient, but is sufficient to prevent any widespread catabolism long enough until the patient is discharged or transferred. You are disappointed that the CPO does not appreciate the importance of your work at the hospital, but you have read the published literature about the metabolic needs of hospitalized patients and the evidence does indeed support a more standardized approach unless the patient is on TPN long-term (weeks/months/years). With this new program, you can potentially stop spending any time on TPN formulations, along with everyone else on the nutritional team, except for the prescribing doctor and the person who enters patient parameters into the program.

You believe that many on the nutrition team will not like this progress and might feel offended that they are being replaced by a program.

Case Question/Instructions

How should you approach the process to adopt the new program and educate the nutritional team and the affected pharmacy staff?

Subcategory: Self-Development

Chapter 2: Transformation

Case #29: Dissent in the Department

You are the Pharmacist in Charge of a pharmacy that is badly split and deeply emotionally invested about how to comply with the Board of Pharmacy rules on sterile compounding. Specifically, the policies and procedures described in the subsection on policies and beyond use dating. You have to get the team to agree on the plan of action, because your annual self-inspection form is due in one month and you have reason to suspect the Board will perform an on-site inspection on or about that time. You definitely feel that you are under the gun, but you are hesitant to simply make executive decision because you are concerned that you will disenfranchise staff that disagree with you.

Case Question/Instructions

What should you do next? So that this problem never occurs again, what would a long-term solution to this problem look like? Write your paper to solve this case, making sure you follow the directions provided by your instructor, and ensure that your paper provides all necessary information outlined in the assignment.

Case #30: Options for the Emergency Department

You have recently been hired as Pharmacy Director of a small rural community hospital. Your hospital has an emergency department that is open 24/7. The retail pharmacies are open seven days per week, but they stay open no later than 9PM on weekdays and only 6PM on weekends. Your inpatient pharmacy is staffed 24/7, but during the night shift, you only have a single pharmacist on duty. This pharmacist's job is to deliver care to patients in the hospital overnight. Your pharmacy does no outpatient prescription dispensing whatsoever.

When introduced to the Service Chief from the emergency department (ED), he says that he wants to set up an appointment with you to figure out how to give medication to patients discharged from his ED late at night: "Enough medication to last them through the night until retail pharmacies open up the next day." He states that he thinks there are rules provided by the Board of Pharmacy that allow physicians to dispense. He wants you to look them up and help him figure this out.

During your next meeting with your boss, the hospital CEO, she says pretty much the same thing. She, however, suggests that you use your night shift pharmacist to perform the late-night prescription dispensing. She says that she feels that the volume would be low enough for the night shift pharmacist to handle it along with the current inpatient activities. She directs you to come to the next Medical Executive Committee meeting, scheduled three weeks from now, with a proposal to start the new service along with cost projections for each option you present.

Case Question/Instructions

What do you recommend at the next Medical Executive Committee meeting? What data or other evidence do you have to support your recommendation?

Case #31: Harvoni®

You are Jennifer, a newly hired pharmacist for Standard Health, which is a privately owned health insurance company in the metro area. As a member of the Drug Information Services (DIS) department, your job is to help the company make policy decisions regarding drug coverage of people who buy your insurance plan. Your company is small. You cover about 200,000 members, mostly in the metro proper. Your company is looking to expand and is marketing to some of the big employers in the area.

You joined Standard Health in part because you felt the company was poised for rapid growth in the near future. You learned during the interview process that Standard Health was very successful in the state insurance exchange, landing new members with low-cost coverage. Even though the new members are disproportionately lower income, you were still impressed that the company learned a lot about how to compete in the marketplace and succeed and grow in the future. You are optimistic that Standard Health will break into the big employer market in the state and start covering the employees of big employers very soon.

The Director of the DIS department, Rick, approached you recently with an important project. Your department is small (for now). Only five pharmacists make up the department. The other four (which includes Rick) are busy with other work. Rick asks you to research a new drug on the market, Harvoni®. Does it make economic sense for us to cover prescriptions written for this drug on our insurance plan? You gladly accepted this project and are flattered that Rick trusts you enough for this work.

You do some fast research and quick calculations. Harvoni® has recently been approved by the FDA to treat Hepatitis C. It is highly effective against this virus that kills tens of thousands of Americans each year. It is horribly expensive! A typical 12-week course of therapy is almost $100,000! You check your company's records and note that your membership has about 2,000 members with the diagnosis of Hepatitis C. If they all get prescriptions for Harvoni®, it would cost your company 200 million dollars! That would surely bankrupt Standard Health! But not covering Harvoni® seems exceptionally cold and unreasonable too.

Case Question/Instructions

What is your recommendation to Rick and the Medical Executive team of Standard Health?

Case #32: Root Cause Analysis

Your name is Karina and you work in a large urban inpatient pharmacy. You graduated pharmacy school about three years ago and this is your first job out of school. You have been gaining loads of valuable clinical skills since graduation, which improves your ability to deliver great care and builds your self-confidence. However, the job remains demanding and requires you to make important care decisions quickly. There are times you feel forced to make hasty clinical decisions and recommendations to medical staff because of the volume of work you are expected to accomplish before the end of your shift. This makes you nervous. It seems that all the other pharmacists survive this nerve-wracking way to practice pharmacy. You have indeed developed loads of advanced clinical skills since graduation and the occasional nervousness you experience is probably nothing more than you still being relatively green in your profession when compared to the other pharmacists in your department. You hope that in the coming months and years, you will get over this sense of impending doom that you occasionally experience.

Next month the hospital is implementing an upgraded computer system that will require doctors and other prescribers to enter orders into the computer instead of writing them out on paper on the patient's chart. You and the rest of the pharmacists feel that this is good for patient safety, and might even give all pharmacists a few extra minutes every day to accomplish all their work. According to the policies that support the new computer system, verbal and phone orders from MDs are forbidden, except when the doctor is out of the hospital and away from the computer system, or occasionally in the case of an authentic clinical emergency where the doctor can't take time to enter the order. This new policy is reassuring to you, since many medication errors are attributed to simple transcription errors when the doctor gives a verbal or phone order.

You are now a month into the new computer system. The doctors are very upset as a group. Many individual doctors have complained to you (and your pharmacist colleagues) that it takes too long for them to click through so many screens and system alerts to enter an order. Many

Chapter 2: Transformation

doctors have resorted to issuing verbal and phone orders in an apparent violation of policy. This puts you and your colleagues in an awkward position. Some doctors are even barking out verbal orders to you as the elevator doors are closing. You and your colleagues have complained to your department Director who assures all of you that she is working on the issue with a variety of hospital leaders, but the resolution to this will take time, since verbal orders are still allowed under certain circumstances.

You took a verbal order from a doctor last week to begin a vancomycin IV on a patient and the patient got too much drug, suffered renal damage, and eventually died. You feel terrible! The prescribing doctor is angry and tells you (privately) that he is disappointed in you because you didn't order the usual and customary peaks and troughs for the drug. You reply, "But you didn't order them doctor!" His reply is that it makes no difference, a "good" pharmacist knows to monitor dangerous drugs closely and would have ordered the labs regardless. Wow, that was very hurtful comment, but you know that the doctor is just trying to cover his own behavior. There is no reason to get into an argument with the doctor about this now. An argumentative debate with this doctor at this time will not help the patient, their family, or the underlying problem (verbal orders). Later that day you are informed that this error is being classified as a sentinel event and that there will be a Root Cause Analysis held the next day and you are expected to attend. You think to yourself, "a root what?!"

Case Question/Instructions

What do you do to prepare for this meeting tomorrow? What will be your message to the team during the Root Cause Analysis?

Case #33: The Law Beats Policy Every Time

You are Kevin, the Pharmacist in Charge at a local outpatient pharmacy that is part of a larger grocery store chain. Your store is in a rural conservative community. Your pharmacy is open 16 hours a day, 7 days a week. You have a small staff of pharmacists and techs that work with you to staff the store. Alyana is one of the pharmacists on your team that works mostly the evening and weekend shifts. She is a good pharmacist with approximately three years of experience in this pharmacy. Alyana is about 30 years old. She is a single mother of a grade school-aged son. You and Alyana have a good working relationship.

You know only a little about Alyana's personal life. You know that Alyana went through a difficult divorce a few years ago. Her husband was accused, arrested, but never convicted of domestic abuse. Alyana privately shared with you that her husband beat her on several occasions and that is why she eventually divorced him. Alyana explained to you that she shares custody of her son with her ex-husband and that, while the continued relationship with her ex is stressful, it is the court ruling and she is nothing if not a law-abiding citizen. She puts up with the hostility she says her husband doles out and she honors the custody agreement. Through all these difficult transitions in her personal life, Alyana has remained highly professional at work. She hardly missed any days on duty and she successfully keeps her personal life at home when she reports to work. You feel empathy towards Alyana and you are immensely thankful that Alyana is dealing with her personal life so professionally. Her personal travails are never the source of gossip or rumors in the pharmacy or in the grocery store, and that is exactly how you want it to remain. You have never had to counsel, coach, or discipline Alyana about any work performance issues or customer satisfaction complaints. Through it all, you have found Alyana a level-headed, mature, even-tempered professional. You secretly wish more of your employees had these same personality traits.

One day, Alyana reports to work on time and is outside your office putting her personal items into her locker. You greet each other as usual. As Alyana puts her bag into her locker, you hear a loud clunk against the thin sheet metal locker. You jokingly ask Alyana if she has bricks in her bag and Alyana casually replies, "No, just my gun." You stop, and your mind begins to race. Alyana finishes getting ready for her shift, closes and locks her locker door and walks out into the pharmacy to begin her shift.

You are startled! A gun in your pharmacy? How many ways could this go wrong? You consider the warning label on the front door of the store that says that no weapons are allowed inside. You ask Alyana to step into your office, and ask her about the gun. Alyana is very casual about it. She says that she has a lawful conceal/carry gun permit and that, given the history with her ex-husband, she carries it for protection. You ask her to remove the gun from her locker and put it in her car or take it home, since the store does not allow any weapons on their property. Alyana seems surprised. "Kevin, I've been carrying the gun for two years now, safely and legally. There has never been a problem. I lock it up in my locker when at work and have never removed it from my locker during my shifts—and don't ever intend to." Alyana goes on to say that she knows the pharmacies within the chain of grocery stores have their own set of policies (because she checked it out two years ago) and there is no rule against guns in the pharmacy. Alyana states, "The law trumps policy every time." Alyana refuses to remove her gun and put it in her car: "It could get stolen, and furthermore the parking lot is grocery store property, so having it in the car creates another problem." You must agree with her logic, but inform her that you will have to take the issue up the chain of command with the pharmacy Regional Director and pharmacy human resources department.

Several days later you get a call from your boss. The boss agrees that there is no policy against carrying a concealed weapon in any of their pharmacies, but he thinks it is a bad idea and tells you to get Alyana to remove the weapon immediately. You object: "I think she will quit and perhaps file some sort of legal action against me for infringing on her right to carry a gun." The boss is unmoved. "If she quits, she quits. I do not want any weapons in any of my pharmacies and I will be writing a policy about this soon."

What do you say to Alyana? You don't want to simply do what your boss says and lose her. She is a good pharmacist and you and everyone else would have to work extra shifts and lots of overtime until her replacement is hired and trained. That is not a good outcome for anyone.

Case Question/Instructions

What should you do next? So that this problem never occurs again, what would a long-term solution to this problem look like? Write your paper to solve this case, making sure you follow the directions provided by your instructor, and ensure that your paper provides all necessary information outlined in the assignment.

Case #34: Fix It!

Your name is Charlie. You have recently been promoted to district manager of 38 retail pharmacies, part of a nationally known chain of retail drug stores. Most are located in affluent suburbs. A few pharmacies are located in urban areas inside or next to medical clinics serving the poor and underserved citizens. One of the first activities as district manager is to visit each pharmacy you are responsible for and talk with the Pharmacist in Charge and staff about issues important to them. You want pharmacy staff to know you as a leader who cares and listens.

Today you are visiting one of your pharmacies on State Ave. It is in an older and low-income neighborhood with more than its fair share of crime. The pharmacy has reinforced security. It has cameras everywhere, numerous burglar and panic alarms, reinforced metal doors, and wrought iron bars on the windows. The pharmacy section of the store is behind bullet-proof glass and doors. Security guards constantly wander up and down the store aisles to deter shoplifting and/or call police if anything unlawful occurs in the store. There is only curbside parking on the street in front of the pharmacy for patients and customers. Graffiti and litter (including used needles and condoms) are chronic problems on and around the exterior of the building. Despite these economic challenges, the pharmacy meets its modest budgetary goals every year. The pharmacy staff is mostly experienced and live in or around the neighborhood and want to help underserved friends and neighbors living in the area. You and the home office want this pharmacy to stay alive even though it would probably be easier and more profitable to move it out to the suburbs. You and your company take pride in keeping this store afloat since it is a concrete expression of your company's commitment to serve people from all walks of life and every economic background.

You are meeting with Jennifer, the Pharmacist in Charge, and she is going through a list of issues she and her staff want help with:

- High-crime neighborhood: several staff have been mugged going to and from work.
- Theft inside the pharmacy is commonplace and cuts into the economic survivability of the store.
- Robberies and burglaries of the prescription area occur a couple of times per year.
- Clinical and pharmacy issues with patients are complex and reflect the underserved nature of the citizens of the surrounding neighborhoods. We need more clinically skilled pharmacists or even new grad pharmacists to meet with, talk to, and help patients manage their chronic conditions better.
- The building is old, but it does not have to be dirty: the janitor is absent most days, and when he is here, he just goes out to the curb to smoke or deal drugs or something because he isn't cleaning.
- We need a better and more inclusive system to help indigent patients who have no money get prescription drugs. Otherwise they get really sick or die due to lack of care. It is really depressing for staff to witness.
- Parking costs $15 per day, even at the "cheap" parking lots nearby; you must do something about the parking for staff.

As you listen to the concerns, you remind yourself how important it is for this store to succeed and for the staff to feel that they are part of something special, not part of a war-zone.

Case Question/Instructions

How should you approach the list of concerns?

Case #35: Controlled Substance Diversion—Loss Prevention

You are a Director of Pharmacy at Universal Health's largest medical center hospital. At a professional meeting you are talking to your colleague from your competitor hospital and find that they have been fined 3 million dollars by the DEA for drug diversion from their Pyxis machines. He is concerned that he will be fired.

You know that your pharmacy is using the same policies and procedures as that institution, because you worked with your friend to write them together. Current Pyxis access monitoring reports are focused on monitoring individual practitioner interactions with the dispensing device. Your system does not track trends or patterns over multiple machines by either discipline or practitioner. You are concerned that if you were audited by the DEA, they would find the same problems at Universal Health.

Case Question/Instructions

What should you do next? So that this problem never occurs again, what would a long-term solution to this problem look like? Write your paper to solve this case, making sure you follow the directions provided by your instructor, and ensure that your paper provides all necessary information outlined in the assignment.

Case #36: What is USP 797?

Your name is Ahmad and you have been recently hired by Standard Medical Center as their Director of Pharmacy. As a fairly recent grad from pharmacy school, this new role for you is a promotion from your prior position as a night shift staff pharmacist from a hospital in another city. You are appropriately proud of your achievement and anxious to get started in your new job. During your first meeting with your new boss, the CEO of the hospital, Randy, he asks you what you know about United States Pharmacopeia (USP) Chapter 797 and if we (the hospital) are compliant with it. You respond with a very high-level description of the requirements of the chapter, but you inform Randy that you will have to assess your department's current status before you can answer the "compliance" question. Randy understands and asks you to come back to him at your next meeting (one month) and not only provide him with current level of compliance, but if you find the pharmacy deficient with the requirements, a high-level plan, time line and ballpark costs to gain compliance.

During the next week in the department, you find that the pharmacy is not compliant with the requirements in USP Chapter 797. Your department has a laminar flow hood in a low-traffic area of the department, but there are no other systems in place that are required by the USP. You check both the previous Board of Pharmacy inspection form and the last inspection from The Joint Commission (TJC). Both inspections were around three years ago. You note in their reports that both agencies noted the gap in compliance and that both agencies required a plan to gain compliance before their next inspection. You check your predecessor's files for steps taken to gain compliance and find basically nothing. This is bad news. Both the TJC and BoP could be back to inspect at any time and you need a detailed plan approved by the hospital board to gain compliance. You'd better advise Randy at your next meeting about this and let him know what it will take to get compliant with the requirements.

Happily, you have a staff in your pharmacy that understands and accepts the need for change and compliance. The prior boss just never took the requirements seriously and therefore nothing was changed to gain compliance. The staff are ready and able to help.

Case Question/Instructions

What should you do next? So that this problem never occurs again, what would a long-term solution to this problem look like? Write your paper to solve this case, making sure you follow the directions provided by your instructor, and ensure that your paper provides all necessary information outlined in the assignment.

Chapter 3: Execution

Subcategory: Accountability

Chapter 3: Execution

Case #37: Coworker Diversion

You are the Pharmacist in Charge at a chain supermarket retail pharmacy. Over the last two months, you have received three complaints from customers that their prescription for controlled substances was short around two to five pills. Two prescriptions were for hydrocodone, and one for oxycodone. Your staff is small, only three pharmacists and four technicians in your pharmacy (including you). One technician and one pharmacist (not you) were involved in preparing the prescription for all three complaints. Not related to these events, you remember hearing a story a year or so ago from one of your colleagues about a pharmacy downstate that fired their Pharmacist in Charge due to loss of controlled substance inventory. Now, just last week, your monthly Schedule 2 Controlled Substance (CII) inventory reconciliation turned up five short of fentanyl patches. You have a very busy pharmacy and all these losses combined add up to 0.03% of all CII doses dispensed in one month of normal business. Despite efforts to locate missing patches, no explanation or reason for the shortage is evident. You begin to suspect that someone on your staff might be diverting inventory.

Case Question/Instructions

What is your plan to stop inventory shrinkage? So that this problem never occurs again, what would a long-term solution to this problem look like? Write your paper to solve this case, making sure you follow the directions provided by your instructor, and ensure that your paper provides all necessary information outlined in the assignment.

Case #38: The Board Says NO!

You are the newly hired Pharmacist in Charge at a small rural hospital pharmacy. Your staff is small: three full-time technicians and two full-time pharmacists (one of whom is you). You took this job in part because you wanted to work in a small, close-knit team doing important work. As you are becoming familiar with the procedures of the department, your partner pharmacist Rusty comes to you in private. He says that the pharmacy techs refill the automated dispensing cabinets around the hospital and attached nursing home every day and their work is not double-checked. He says that is against pharmacy laws and regulations. You reply that the barcode scanning system double-checks each med and dose prior to administration and that the techs are not dispensing to the patient, but to other licensed caregivers (registered nurses and occasionally MDs), so no big deal. The process is just like the process used in the larger hospital from which you were just recruited, and they passed Board inspection just five months ago. Rusty is not convinced. You ask Rusty to relax and inform him that you will consider his concern as you continue your orientation.

Six months later, your orientation is long since complete. You did consider Rusty's concern and felt comfortable with your prior opinion. The techs do a great job refilling the cabinets accurately. You have spot-checked them periodically and they have been refilled 100% accurately. You are the pharmacist accountable for compliance with Board rules. You elected to make no changes. Since your schedule rarely allows for you and Rusty to work at the same time, you have not had a chance to talk to him about your decision. The few minutes per week that you are face to face with him, you are both busy sharing shift information and other important clinical patient information. You simply forget to talk to Rusty about his concern expressed six months ago. He has never brought it up again. By now, you reckon this issue is resolved.

In the seventh month of your employment, Rusty comes in on his day off to talk to you. He reminds you of his expressed concern seven months ago during your orientation and says that he feels like you ignored him. Then he states that he contacted the Board of Pharmacy and asked them about the issue and he feels that he is right, it is illegal for our techs to refill the machines without a pharmacist double check. He says that we need to change our process quickly, because the inspector he talked to seemed surprised that you let the techs refill the machines without a double check and indicated that he would have to come see for himself. Rusty states that he feels that the inspector will be here soon to see for himself. You asked Rusty why he would not come to you first before going to the Board of Pharmacy? He says he did and that you ignored him. He goes on to say that his license is "on the line" too and that the Board's mission is public safety. He says that the Board of Pharmacy seeks input, concerns, and complaints from all state residents, not just Pharmacists in Charge.

Case Question/Instructions

What do you do about Rusty's action and the fact that the Board may be coming soon to inspect? So that this problem never occurs again, what would a long-term solution to this problem look like? Write your paper to solve this case, making sure you follow the directions provided by your instructor, and ensure that your paper provides all necessary information outlined in the assignment.

Case #39: Résumé Discrepancy

Your name is Quintin. You are the owner of Universal Drugs in a small rural town. You also own and manage State Drugs, which is a very busy pharmacy in a larger community 35 miles away from Universal Drugs. State Drugs is located in a suburb of a larger city and must compete with some big-box pharmacies. These big-box stores have occasionally used some pretty aggressive pricing tactics to wrestle patients away from State Drugs. Although you have figured out how to compete with the grocery store and big-box pharmacies at State Drugs, Universal Drugs has had no pressure and has enjoyed growing prescription volume over the last few years. Now you hear that one big-box chain pharmacy is planning to build a new pharmacy just three blocks from Universal Drugs. It is scheduled to open in nine months. Your Pharmacy Manager at Universal Drugs is Dave. Dave has never competed with big chain stores before and none of the staff pharmacists have either. You lack faith in Dave's ability to lead Universal Drugs through the necessary changes in operations to successfully compete with the big-box pharmacies. You personally don't have the bandwidth to micromanage Dave through the challenging times ahead. Therefore, you have a talk with Dave and you both agree that his job will soon change drastically and become a position that is very different. You spell out clearly all the stresses and challenges in Dave's future if he stays. This is not what Dave signed up for. You two eventually agree to part amicably so that you can hire someone to manage Universal Drugs through some tough times ahead. To acknowledge Dave's past contributions, you offer Dave a generous severance package and Dave agrees to stay on for up to six months to help you select and train the next manager.

Sometime later, you plan to interview Brandi for the manager of Universal Drugs position. You selected her for interview based in part on her résumé. She worked in a large metropolitan area for the same large chain that will be opening next to Universal Drugs. Brandi listed management experience there as part of her work history. You also selected her for interview because Dave and two other pharmacists at Universal Drugs know Brandi from school and recommend her. Her phone interview was favorable too. The next step will be for Brandi to come for a face-to-face interview with you and your team. Brandi gave you permission to contact several references prior to the face-to-face interview. You contacted Nicole, one of Brandi's pharmacist coworkers at the big-box pharmacy where she previously worked. Nicole confirms everything Brandi states in her résumé, except for the following;

Brandi was an interim manager with the big-box store for six weeks only. That was not stated in her résumé or revealed in your phone interview with her.

Brandi's résumé states that the time worked at the competitor chain was 3 years and 4 months (40 months). Nicole says that she clearly remembers when Brandi started work because she trained Brandi after her hire. Nicole says that Brandi worked at this store for 34 months.

Chapter 3: Execution

Case Question/Instructions

What should you do next? So that this problem never occurs again, what would a long-term solution to this problem look like? Write your paper to solve this case, making sure you follow the directions provided by your instructor, and ensure that your paper provides all necessary information outlined in the assignment.

Case #40: Threat of Violence

You are Steve; a pharmacist who lives and works in a small community. Being one of only two pharmacies in the community, it can get super busy and there is a high volume of prescriptions that are filled and dispensed each day. You generally enjoy your coworkers and regular customers, many of which refer to you by your first name.

Last month, you received a new prescription for paroxetine for Johnny, a seventeen-year-old who picks up his own prescriptions. According to your information system, at the time, Johnny was taking the SSRI sertraline to manage his depression—you remember having to call his doctor for verification that he would only be taking the new antidepressant paroxetine and not both agents together. During that call, Johnny's doctor told you that the sertraline was not effective for him anymore and to go ahead and discontinue that prescription in the system; Johnny would be trying the paroxetine for at least two months to see if that would work better for him.

When Johnny picked up the paroxetine prescription for the first time last month, he did not look too good. When you were counseling him on the new medication, he mentioned that he was hoping this new medication would work better because he has been feeling so depressed that he didn't even know how he talked to his doctor about it. He said he was falling behind at school, unable to sleep right, and often wouldn't even bother to get up in the morning.

You've known Johnny and his family since Johnny was 10 years old; he used to be such a happy child, but since his father passed away two years ago, he hasn't been the same. He became extremely withdrawn, and his mother has mentioned in the past that he has had violent bursts of anger, and just couldn't cope with things very well. You have tried to be available to talk to either of them when they come into the pharmacy, and it seemed to help Johnny a little to have someone to talk to.

Johnny is due to come in and pick up the second month's supply of his paroxetine, and you're curious to see if he is feeling better. Shortly after high school lets out, you see Johnny enter the pharmacy and immediately notice he looks upset, frustrated, and angry.

"Hey Johnny, how are you doing?" you ask.

"Horrible," Johnny blurts out, "I'm so mad. Things are messed up at school, I'm so pissed off!"

"What do you mean? Do you want to talk about it?"

"No! I just need to pick up this medication! I have to go home and get some stuff done," he says, angrily.

As Johnny walks out of the pharmacy, he is still talking to himself in an angry tone, "Sometimes I wish I never existed. And I wish that school never existed! Things would be so much better if it was burned to the ground!" Johnny continues just loud enough that you can make out what he is saying as he leaves, before you can say anything else.

SLAM goes the door!

Case Question/Instructions

What should you do next? Write your paper to solve this case, making sure you follow the directions provided by your instructor, and ensure that your paper provides all necessary information outlined in the assignment.

Case #41: Medication Error

As the manager of a retail pharmacy, you receive a call from the mother of one of your patients stating that she had to take her daughter to the emergency department for a severe drug reaction due to an Augmentin Liquid prescription that your pharmacy filled. You note that there is an amoxicillin allergy noted in her profile. In reviewing the prescription, you find that your best friend on the staff filled the prescription but bypassed the usage warning when the system alerted them.

Case Question/Instructions

What should you do next? So that this problem never occurs again, what would a long-term solution to this problem look like? Write your paper to solve this case, making sure you follow the directions provided by your instructor, and ensure that your paper provides all necessary information outlined in the assignment.

Case #42: Vaccine Expiration and Recall

You work as a pharmacist at Standard Health Systems, and have recently discovered that one of your staff pharmacists administered an outdated rabies vaccine to one of the pharmacy's patients. After recognizing the error, you would like to communicate it to fellow pharmacists and staff as a teachable moment. To add to the issue, the rabies vaccine administered to the patient was recalled earlier this year, but unfortunately not pulled from the shelf.

Case Question/Instructions

What do you do now? So that this problem never occurs again, what would a long-term solution to this problem look like? Write your paper to solve this case, making sure you follow the directions provided by your instructor, and ensure that your paper provides all necessary information outlined in the assignment.

Case #43: Shoo-in

You are Becky, a recent pharmacy graduate working in a downtown retail pharmacy. This is a privately owned, independent chain of five stores. You meet with the owner, Carl, a couple of times, one on one. You let Carl know that you want to be promoted to Pharmacist in Charge (PIC) at one of his stores when you're ready and have sufficient experience. Carl registers your ambition. Since Carl is happy with how his current PICs are performing, he encourages you to observe and get mentoring from your store's PIC, as well as the PICs in the other stores.

Several years go by and you observe that one of the unique skillsets a PIC must have is being able to solve problems on the fly, sometimes multiple problems at the same time! You have paid particular attention to the problem-solving techniques used by your own PIC and, when you work in the other stores, how other PICs solve problems in their stores. You ask the PIC in your primary store to allow you some practice at problem solving and your PIC is helpful, referring day-to-day problems to you on several occasions. You are clumsy at first, but become better and more skillful at problem solving with experience.

The day comes that a PIC in one of the other stores resigns and you apply for the job. Your current PIC encourages you, and tells you she will put in a good word with Carl for you. You are excited and think you are a shoo-in for the job. You interview well; you think you've "nailed it!" You then find out that a 63-year-old white male, Ben, got the job. A man who has no experience with independent retail pharmacies. You approach Carl and ask why you didn't get the job. Carl says that he gave the job to Ben because he is a member of a protected class of citizens and he doesn't want to get sued for discrimination if he gives the job to anyone else.

Chapter 3: Execution

Case Question/Instructions

What do you do next? So that this problem never occurs again, what would a long-term solution to this problem look like? Write your paper to solve this case, making sure you follow the directions provided by your instructor, and ensure that your paper provides all necessary information outlined in the assignment.

Case #44: Patient Privacy

You are a pharmacist at an inpatient hospital pharmacy. You just learned that your ex-spouse is in the hospital and is in a very serious condition. You are on duty and assigned to the intensive care ward where your ex-spouse is located. You monitor your ex's clinical condition as part of your job and fulfill all the duties related to delivering the appropriate pharmaceutical care she needs to aid in her recovery. During your break you take the time to log into the information system to look over your ex's history and physical in the medical record, because you still care and are genuinely curious about what happened. Later that day, your ex-mother-in-law calls you and starts asking you all sorts of questions in a frantic frame of mind. "Please help me! The doctors are confusing me!" You know all the answers to your ex-mother-in-law's questions and you genuinely want to help ease her mind.

Case Question/Instructions

What do you do?

SUBCATEGORY: CHANGE LEADERSHIP

Chapter 3: Execution

Case #45: My U-500 Insulin

A diabetic patient is admitted for an elective surgery to the hospital where you work as a staff pharmacist. Among the medications noted on her admission medication reconciliation is insulin, 80 units injected subcutaneously morning and evening. The patient has brought her own insulin with her, a vial of Humulin R 500U/ml, and wants to continue to use this during her stay in the hospital. She experiences pain on injection when the injection is over 0.5 ml volume. She will be discharged on the U-500 dosage after the surgery. The hospital formulary uses a standardized U-100 dose for all insulin dosing. You check your policy manual, and there is no direction about how to process patient requests to use their own medication while hospitalized.

The Nursing Supervisor comes to you, since you are on the patient's care team, and expresses her concern for the potential for serious medication errors if the concentrated U-500 is present in the general nursing unit. She tells you to store the patient's U-500 insulin in the pharmacy until the patient is discharged, and have the patient use the U-100 insulin that is stocked in the Pyxis machines on the floor.

Case Question/Instructions

What should you do to appropriately manage this person's diabetes during her stay in the hospital? So that this problem never occurs again, what would a long-term solution to this problem look like? Write your paper to solve this case, making sure you follow the directions provided by your instructor, and ensure that your paper provides all necessary information outlined in the assignment.

Case #46: Employer Hiring Practices

You, Shannon, are a pharmacist on a team that has been gathered to perform job interviews and help select the best candidate to join your department. LaDonna is the hiring manager and her heritage is what many would describe as "African American." The hiring manager makes the hiring decisions. Based on your interview questions and scores, the best and highest scoring candidate is Hope. Her heritage would be what many describe as "Native American." LaDonna holds a very open and transparent interview process. The interview team shares interview scores, and thoughts and comments about each candidate. A majority of the team feel that, based on score alone, Hope should be offered the job. About half of the team feels that Hope's personality would fit nicely with the rest of the department. The other half of the team doesn't comment on "fit" one way or another. After gathering input from the entire team, including you, LaDonna makes the following summary comments:

"Thank you all for your input. Hope did score the highest of all the candidates. I'm concerned that Hope will be a poor personality fit with our department. We need new people who will work hard and are highly dependable. I'm not so sure that Hope has this work ethic. Based on her answers to interview questions, I think Hope comes from a very low socio-economic situation. She didn't reveal any moral center in her answers. She didn't describe any standards of behaviors that she admires or seeks to emulate. We know that alcoholism, drug abuse, and employee theft occur at high rates among people with a low socioeconomic upbringing. All pharmacies are targets for robbery and theft. We have lots of money and drugs that many people would love to steal from us. I don't need the risk that I think Hope represents. We don't need that risk. I am not going to offer our job to any of the candidates and bring in another group of applicants next month."

No one expresses support for LaDonna's decision. No one objects either.

Later, in private, you ask LaDonna what evidence she has that Hope might have alcoholism, or tendency toward criminal behaviors? LaDonna responds, "Read the newspapers, it's common knowledge."

Case Question/Instructions

What should you do next? So that this problem never occurs again, what would a long-term solution to this problem look like? Write your paper to solve this case, making sure you follow the directions provided by your instructor, and ensure that your paper provides all necessary information outlined in the assignment.

Case #47: Personal Property

You are an inpatient pharmacist who works in a hospital that securely stores any valuables patients bring in when they are admitted. Typically, this includes money, jewelry, watches, or laptops/devices that the patient won't use while in the hospital. Personal valuables are usually kept in a locked safe or locker in the Admitting Department. Frequently patients bring in all their medications too. Patients do this often, so doctors and nurses can see what they are taking. If they don't have family or friends to take the meds back home, the hospital will store personal medications in the inpatient pharmacy and, like other personal valuables, return them when the patient is discharged.

One day you are called by a patient's nurse to take personal medications for safekeeping in the pharmacy. You collect the bag and as you are logging them into the system, as required by policy, you see a small, clear plastic baggie of white powder, and insulin syringes. One of the syringes is partially filled with clear red/pinkish liquid. The syringe tip is capped. You look up the patient's medical record and he is not diabetic nor has never been prescribed insulin or any other self-injected medication. In fact, you notice that the reason for the patient's admission to the hospital is a drug overdose of opiate, maybe heroin. The diagnosis is confirmed when you notice when in the hospital's emergency department, the patient coded and was instantly resuscitated by the administration of naloxone. You conclude that an opiate (probably heroin) is in the bag of powder and liquefied in the partial syringe. The pinkish color to the liquid in the syringe is probably the patient's blood. You log the substance into the pharmacy system as unknown ("illicit injectable opiate" is not an option on the menu). You feel uncomfortable storing an illicit (probably Schedule 1) controlled substance in the pharmacy. You feel even less comfortable returning the drug to the patient upon discharge. Later that day, you check policy and it says that we (the hospital) return all personal property (including personal drugs) to the patient upon discharge. You check with the Pharmacy Manager who reinforces this policy by saying that we (the hospital) don't confiscate personal property even if we feel it might be the best thing to do for the patient. Your boss goes on to say that we (the hospital) provide care to anyone who seeks it without prejudice. Your boss asks you to keep the unknown substance in the pharmacy and to return it when the patient is discharged. You feel this is not right and that for the patient's overall health, the illicit drug should be destroyed and not returned to the patient.

Case Question/Instructions

What should you do next? So that this problem never occurs again, what would a long-term solution to this problem look like? Write your paper to solve this case, making sure you follow the directions provided by your instructor, and ensure that your paper provides all necessary information outlined in the assignment.

Case #48: Unwanted Drugs

Your name is Melody and you recently graduated from pharmacy school and moved to a lovely rural community, where you accepted a job as a pharmacist in the local pharmacy. After a few weeks on the job, as you explore the back of the pharmacy for storage space for some new compounding equipment, you run across a banker's box of partially filled prescription vials

Chapter 3: Execution

from a wide variety of pharmacies from the surrounding region. You examine the labels on the vials and note that most of the drugs were dispensed a year or more ago. Some are controlled substances; however, most are not. You ask your coworker pharmacist John what the box of drugs represents. John says that the owner has provided the community a service to accept expired and unwanted drugs from consumers, typically after the patient has died or no longer needs them. John says that many members of the community don't like flushing drugs in the sewer system as it poisons local water sources. The owner collects unwanted prescription drugs, free of charge, and when the box fills up he incinerates the box of drugs at local incinerator. There are no records or permits kept by the pharmacy. The owner says the drugs are no longer wanted, so no records are needed, he says he started up this service many years ago because his customers want to destroy unwanted drugs in a responsible manner, particularly controlled substances to keep them "off the street." You have vague recollections that there are both state and federal laws and rules that pertain to destruction of prescription drugs and you fear that what the owner is doing might be in violation of one or more rules or laws.

Case Question/Instructions

What should you do next? So that this problem never occurs again, what would a long-term solution to this problem look like? Write your paper to solve this case, making sure you follow the directions provided by your instructor, and ensure that your paper provides all necessary information outlined in the assignment.

Subcategory: Organizational Awareness

Chapter 3: Execution

Case #49: Delegation and Allocation of Resources

You are the Pharmacist in Charge. You and your team are in the midst of a massive surge in prescription volume. Customers are restless and waiting impatiently. Some on your team are working madly (maybe recklessly), others are plodding along doing their work and not helping the team get through the surge. They are doing their assigned work well enough, but basically just watching their coworkers suffer through the massive workload.

Case Question/Instructions

What should you do next? So that this problem never occurs again, what would a long-term solution to this problem look like? Write your paper to solve this case, making sure you follow the directions provided by your instructor, and ensure that your paper provides all necessary information outlined in the assignment.

Case #50: An FTE is Not Always an FTE

You are the Manager of a long-term care (LTC) pharmacy. You were hired into this position one year ago and it is your first management job. You are proud of your career advancements since graduation and you are indeed on track with the professional development plan you made prior to graduating. You want to express your thanks and repay your bosses by expanding your department's services, aimed at improving quality of life experiences for the residents at your client LTC facilities. You propose a new pain control service you learned about in one of your APPE (Advanced Pharmacy Practice Experience) rotations prior to graduation. You feel the new service will control pain better and not "snow" the residents with opiates or other central nervous system depressants. You are confident of the program's potential and you and your staff have done the needed research to convince the decision-makers that this service is worth the 1.4 FTE pharmacists you will need to perform the service. You explain to your boss you need eight hours of work from pain pharmacists per day, seven days a week: $(8 \times 7) \div 40 = 1.4$ FTEs.

You and your pharmacist team do a fantastic job getting approval for the new pain service. It is approved with great fanfare by the medical directors and your boss. Immediately after approval of the service, a small tasteful victory celebration occurs in the pharmacy. Morale in your department is sky-high! Your service is successfully implemented several months later, after hiring and training. Just as you predicted, the residents and nurses and families love the new service. Residents are getting good pain control and are not always sleeping under the influence of opiates. Your quality control metrics are all in line with what you predicted. It is all good.

Then your budget report comes, several months into the new service. You are over budget on your FTEs, starting at the same time you started the new pain service. How can that be? You hired 1.4 FTEs and that is what you scheduled on your department staffing schedule. You go to the LTC pharmacy budget officer and ask for help understanding the report. The budget officer Alexis explains that she increased your budget by 1.4 FTE, but your "burn rate" is more like 1.6 FTEs. How is that?! Alexis points out that you are giving your pain pharmacists paid vacation and sick time, aren't you? "Of course," you reply. Alexis responds, "Well that's non-productive time. I increased your budget by 1.4 total FTEs and you increased your budget by 1.4 productive FTEs. The problem is that you forgot to account for paid non-productive time. Too bad for you. You will need to reduce your staff by roughly 0.2 FTE to stay in budget."

Case Question/Instructions

What should you do next? So that this problem never occurs again, what would a long-term solution to this problem look like? Write your paper to solve this case, making sure you follow the direc-

tions provided by your instructor, and ensure that your paper provides all necessary information outlined in the assignment.

Case #51: Snow Day

It is mid-January and the weather forecast calls for snow flurries with no measurable precipitation. Your pharmacy is scheduled to open the next morning at 9AM. No special staffing plans for tomorrow are needed since the road conditions should be fine.

You wake up the next morning and there is indeed a light accumulation of snow, just as forecasted. The temperature is below freezing, but no matter, there isn't enough snow to make any difference to careful drivers. You get in your car at 8:30 to head to work. During your short commute, you notice your car is slipping a lot. After taking it slowly and safely, you finally make it to work at 8:56 and slide to the front door to open the pharmacy. Two technicians are waiting to be let in. You ask them where the rest of the staff is. They don't know. As soon as you get in the door and turn off the alarms, your phones start ringing. All three of you start triaging the calls. Most are from panicky customers wanting refills before the blizzard hits. Blizzard? One of your techs turns on the store TV. The forecast has changed to an accumulation of up to 10 inches by tonight, with light snow and ice until tonight when the storm hits. Your other tech tells you that the other calls were from the rest of the staff (two pharmacists and one more tech) saying that they can't get to work due to black ice and looming blizzard conditions.

You already have refill calls for 15 prescriptions and the phone is still ringing with more refill requests. Customers are starting to slide in to stock up on prescriptions and other household and food items. Way too much work for you and your two techs. Your two techs are pretty green and are beginning to panic and suggest that you close the pharmacy, so they can go home.

Case Question/Instructions

How should you proceed with organizing your work day with your limited staff? So that this problem never occurs again, what would a long-term solution to this problem look like? Write your paper to solve this case, making sure you follow the directions provided by your instructor, and ensure that your paper provides all necessary information outlined in the assignment.

Case #52: Missing Pharmacy Manager

You work as a staff pharmacist at State retail pharmacy. It is a small chain of independent retail pharmacies. You have seven stores situated in small cities of less than 25,000 residents. The manager of your pharmacy is Carl. Carl is a disaster! Carl is never in the pharmacy for more than a few hours, and on some days, he doesn't show up at all except to open and then to close the pharmacy.

Many times, Carl takes extended lunch breaks and will sometimes come back right before the pharmacy is closing for the night. He claims to be spending time with other outside pharmacy employees such as pharmacists from other stores and Regional Managers, but you (and your coworkers) have never heard any substantiating information to support his claim. Additionally, there have been a few times where you were sure you smelled alcohol on Carl's breath when he came back into the pharmacy, although he did not appear to be impaired.

Carl's lack of presence is a problem as it directly affects patients and your workflow. When Carl is not in the pharmacy and there is no other float pharmacist scheduled, prescription production bottlenecks occur before the final verification step. There have been patients who have not been able to pick up their prescriptions on time and as a result you have lost several of your customers to competing pharmacies.

Carl cares nothing about the pharmacy business and provides absolutely no leadership. When a patient is picking up their medication and it is a new prescription, Carl tells staff to

Chapter 3: Execution

just ask them if they need counseling and if they decline, then don't counsel. Also, there have also been a number of mistakes where customers have received another patient's prescription because Carl put the prescription for patient "A" into the bag for patient "B" during the final steps of the verification process.

Morale is so awful that people are actively seeking other jobs. The entire staff feels that the district management should be told about this situation, but you're not sure where to go or who to talk to.

Case Question/Instructions

What should you do next? What would a long-term solution to this problem look like? Write your paper to solve this case, making sure you follow the directions provided by your instructor, and ensure that your paper provides all necessary information outlined in the assignment.

Case #53: Informal Leader—Not in a Good Way

Your name is Leema and you are the Director of Pharmacy at Standard Medical Center (SMC), in a small rural hospital whose pharmacy is entirely centralized. Your department offers very few clinical services due to limited staff and budget. You have consistently advocated to hospital senior leaders for your department to perform more services, but due to the necessary expansion of staff and services elsewhere in the hospital, each proposal from your department has been denied. You understand the big picture and realize that the hospital has "bigger fish to fry," to borrow a phrase. You are not frustrated. Maybe a bit disappointed, but not frustrated.

Today your new hire, pharmacist Erin, comes to you excited about a conversation she has had with Dr. Turnbull, the hospital's Chief of Staff. You hired Erin away from a state hospital three months ago and since her hire she has performed beautifully. She has developed genuine relationships with you and your staff. Erin seems genuinely happy with her new position at SMC. Erin started her meeting with you very excited about what Dr. Turnbull said. Erin tells you about Dr. Turnbull's vision to start up a pharmacist-based anticoagulation service for hospitalized patients at SMC. You are impressed. You agree that this would be a good service for your department to manage. Because of Erin's experience at the state hospital, you know she is familiar with this kind of service. You ask Erin to describe what it would take to build an anticoagulation service at SMC. Erin answers your question. Basically, it would require you to add two new pharmacist positions and require the development and approval of one or more pharmacy practice agreements with the medical staff. You remember your past experiences with hospital administration. You already know that asking for more pharmacists will be denied. The hospital simply does not have that kind of money laying around. You don't want to discourage or frustrate Erin, but you also don't want to mislead her or give her any false sense of hope.

You give Erin an honest answer about the chances of success, given the current financial pressures on the hospital. You agree to meet with Dr. Turnbull and Erin to discuss his vision, but you make it abundantly clear to Erin that there is little hope for any clinical service at SMC that requires the addition of staff. The next week, before your promised meeting with Erin and Dr. Turnbull, you are in a routine monthly meeting with your boss Sally, the Vice-President of Patient Care Services at SMC. Sally is not happy. Sally tells you that Dr. Turnbull and about half of the medical staff are excited about some plan to create a pharmacist-based anticoagulation service. Sally is concerned about added costs and all the related work to develop such a program, and asks why you haven't come to her to explain this plan for a new pharmacy service? Sally asks you directly, "why did I have to hear about this at Medical Executive Committee meeting, and not directly from you first? I was totally unprepared to respond!" After that unhappy meeting with Sally, you ask some questions and hear from three different doctors that Erin is actively building consensus among the medical staff for the service, to pressure hospital administration into "footing the bill." This is not good. You ask Erin what she knows. Erin openly admits, "Boss, since your hands were tied with hospital administration and they tend to listen to the medical staff, I thought it would be helpful to get the doctors to ask for the service instead of you. That way the hospital would have to say yes if all the doctors wanted it."

Case Question/Instructions

What should you do next? So that this problem never occurs again, what would a long-term solution to this problem look like? Write your paper to solve this case, making sure you follow the directions provided by your instructor, and ensure that your paper provides all necessary information outlined in the assignment.

Case #54: Negotiation and Prioritization of Work

You are Heather, and you have just begun your Post-Graduate Year 2 residency in infectious disease at an academic medical center. Your major project this year will be to redesign the distribution system of intermittent IV antibiotic doses at the hospital. The goals of this project are numerous:

Reduce costs by converting from expensive premixed frozen piggyback antibiotic bags to less expensive "click-on vial" alternatives;

Decrease waste through reduction of expired doses. Design and implement a distribution system that leverages Pyxis dispensing cabinets instead of batch preparation and the cart-fill delivery system currently used;

Develop new extended stability guidelines and workflow processes for pharmacy staff that will support the alternative Pyxis-based distribution system;

Ensure that patient safety is maintained when the alternative distribution system is implemented;

Develop safety, efficiency, and cost metrics with targets for each to measure the success of the newly implemented distribution system;

Develop communication and education plans for pharmacy staff and nursing staff to minimize risk of medication errors.

You are excited about this major project, and confident you can manage all the demands of your upcoming year. About three months into your residency, you are keeping up with your rotations, staffing, and project assignment timelines, although you are working long days and using weekends to stay on track with your numerous responsibilities. In two weeks, a major milestone will be reached with your antibiotic distribution redesign project: the first two med/surg nursing units will pilot the new distribution design. You are madly working to push out your communication and education plan to pharmacy and nursing departments. It's crunch time for the next two or three weeks for sure!

Today at noon, your primary preceptor calls and asks if you can research some alternatives to a sudden and unexpected national shortage of IV ciprofloxacin. The request includes the need to develop a communication plan for medical and nursing staffs. The hospital will run out of IV ciprofloxacin by this coming weekend and the medical and pharmacy staff need to know what clinical alternatives exist until the shortage is over. You want to help. This problem is right up your alley in terms of expertise. But if you divert any time away from your major project, there will be delays to the launch of your pilot, which is scheduled to go in two weeks. You have put too much work into your distribution redesign project and too many people are involved to make any delay in the upcoming pilot palatable for anyone, least of all you. On the other hand, if you don't get involved in the looming shortage of ciprofloxacin, the quality of care delivered to patients might significantly suffer, and that would also be inexcusable on your watch.

Chapter 3: Execution

Case Question/Instructions

What should you do next? So that this problem never occurs again, what would a long-term solution to this problem look like? Write your paper to solve this case, making sure you follow the directions provided by your instructor, and ensure that your paper provides all necessary information outlined in the assignment.

Case #55: Whose FTE Is This Anyway?

Your name is Jenna and you are the Director of Inpatient Pharmacy in a large urban hospital. Your pharmacy operates 24/7 and you have approximately 35 pharmacists and approximately 35 techs who report to you and your administrative team. Just like every other acute care facility in the land, your hospital is in the process of cutting staff wherever possible. Your boss recently asked you for opportunities to cut staff to be more efficient. The objective is not to lay anyone off, but unless the hospital, as a whole, does a better job making existing staff work more efficiently, then layoffs are possible.

You take this challenge to your leadership team. Your Clinical Coordinator, Victoire, suggests cutting two shifts per week devoted to the Infectious Disease (ID) pharmacists and then use those shifts instead to grant more time off for regular staff pharmacists who are being denied their vacation requests too often. Your leadership team likes the concept but asks you to provide some more detail, particularly about the elimination of the ID shifts and the services they provide.

Victoire explains that the ID pharmacists staff their shifts every Wednesday and use their time to look over every patient in the hospital on antibiotics. They look in each patient's chart for any contraindications for the antibiotic the patient is on, like mismatched sensitivity reports, allergies, side effects, etc. The ID pharmacists make their list of suggestions for optimization of antibiotic therapy and give the list to the ID doctor who makes rounds every Wednesday afternoon. Victoire explains that the services provided by the ID pharmacists are not advanced practice stuff and that all staff pharmacists should be doing this service every day, not just two "special pharmacists" on Wednesdays. Victoire suggests that the leadership team (under her guidance) develop a training plan to "spin up" all the staff pharmacists to perform this basic-level antimicrobial stewardship and then use the ID pharmacists as clinical resources for staff pharmacists as needed. When the staff pharmacists are ready to take over the ID duties, then remove the two shifts per week and use the two ID pharmacists to cover more vacation requests. Everyone wins! Victoire thinks it might take the staff pharmacists a couple of months to receive the training and implement the change.

Several weeks later, after you give staff pharmacists the good news about your plan, you are contacted by the Chief of Infectious Disease Service, Dr. Penner. He wants to meet with you right away. He states that he does not believe that just any pharmacist can be trained to provide the ID support the two ID pharmacists offer. You try to explain the intended benefits of the plan including timely (seven days per week) antibiotic optimization recommendations to doctors instead of the one day per week optimization that is currently in place. You explain that no other medical specialty gets the support of "special pharmacists" with extra shifts added to the staffing schedule, so why should ID? You explain that the two pharmacists who provide the valuable ID service to his team are not Board Certified in ID and are "merely" staff pharmacists just like every other pharmacist in your department. You acknowledge that the two "special" pharmacists, through their own initiative, became knowledgeable with antimicrobial stewardship standards and service and that they do a good job, but the fact remains, they have no credentials above or beyond that of any "regular" pharmacist. You explain that if the "special" pharmacists can learn the information it takes to support the ID team, the other pharmacists can too, given the chance.

You both start repeating yourselves with no progress towards resolution. You reach impasse. Your final comment to Dr. Penner is that these FTEs are in the pharmacy budget, so it is your decision, not his.

One day later, your boss demands a meeting with you and he chews you out. "How can you be so stubborn with Dr. Penner?" Once again, you go through the list of benefits and finish your explanation to your boss by saying something like, "I'm only carrying out your direction to operate more efficiently." Your boss seems unmoved and more interested in making Dr. Penner happy than anything else. Your boss requires you to come to the next Pharmacy and Therapeutics committee meeting in two weeks, to explain the details of your antimicrobial stewardship program to the entire committee and why you want to remove the ID pharmacists from their support of the ID department. He tells you that he will invite Dr. Penner and the hospital CEO to attend and listen to your presentation. No pressure!

Case Question/Instructions

What should you do next? So that this problem never occurs again, what would a long-term solution to this problem look like? Write your paper to solve this case, making sure you follow the directions provided by your instructor, and ensure that your paper provides all necessary information outlined in the assignment.

Special Instructions

In addition to all the required elements, your paper will include an explanation about what constitutes a good antimicrobial stewardship program in the USA today and how your plan, as set out in this case, will move your hospital closer to current professional standards for an antimicrobial stewardship program. Your paper should explain in some level of detail how you plan to train all the pharmacists to provide this service and how you plan to change Dr. Penner's mind.

Chapter 4: Ethics

Subcategory: Accountability

Chapter 4: Ethics

Case #56: Poor Medical Practice

You are Barry, an experienced pharmacist in a local retail pharmacy. You have stable clientele and you know most of the doctors who write prescriptions for your patients. You detect that Dr. Jones has a pattern of peculiar prescribing habits. For instance, you know that, on occasion, he writes prescriptions for antibiotics for his patients without seeing them in his office first. He has a few patients for which he writes Schedule 2 Controlled Substance prescriptions regularly for vague clinical reasons and sometimes additional drugs that appear to be contraindicated (i.e. amphetamines and opiates at the same time for the same patient). In general, you find that Dr. Jones engages in these "dubious" prescribing patterns too often for your own comfort. You come to the conclusion that something must be done about Dr. Jones.

Case Question/Instructions

What should you do next? What would a long-term solution to this problem look like? Write your paper to solve this case, making sure you follow the directions provided by your instructor, and ensure that your paper provides all necessary information outlined in the assignment.

Subcategory: Achievement Orientation

Chapter 4: Ethics

Case #57: U.S. Healthcare System and Healthcare Disparities: The Case of No Coverage

It is your first week working as a licensed pharmacist and today is your first Saturday alone. You have one experienced technician working with you. It is late in the day, about 10 minutes to closing time, and a patient comes in with a long list of discharge medications from the nearby hospital. Your technician is able to collect insurance information and this patient is using Medicaid. All of the 10 new discharge medications go through on the insurance except one of the most important ones, the insulin. The insulin is written as the Lantus Solostar Pen. It is denied by the Pharmacy Benefits Manager system, requiring a Prior Authorization.

You call the hospital and they are unable to help with this until Monday and real live people at the insurance company are already gone for the weekend. This patient needs his insulin.

Case Question/Instructions

What should you do next? What would a long-term solution to this problem look like? Write your paper to solve this case, making sure you follow the directions provided by your instructor, and ensure that your paper provides all necessary information outlined in the assignment.

Subcategory: Change Leadership

Chapter 4: Ethics

Case #58: Ethical Dilemma with Drug Abuser

Your name is Sandy and you are a staff pharmacist at a small rural hospital. You graduated from pharmacy school four years ago. Part of your professional development plan is to apply all the tools and skills you learned in leadership courses at school to become a Pharmacy Director at this, or another, hospital. You plan to stay at this, your first job out of school, for three to five years before actively seeking a leadership position. One month ago, you learned that the Director of your pharmacy is planning to retire in the next six months and you would love to apply and be seriously considered for the Director of Pharmacy position. You are actively thinking (almost on a daily basis) how you can distinguish yourself from all the other applicants you anticipate applying for the job. Nothing has come to mind yet but still you contemplate some sort of "home run" you can pull off to demonstrate to hospital leaders that you are the right person for the job once they begin recruitment. In the meantime, you are simply doing your best to be a great clinical pharmacist, delivering great pharmaceutical care on a daily basis.

Today you are working in the emergency department (ED) of the hospital and a 35-year-old patient, Martha Smith, is being treated for a serious infection. You are consulting with the treating ED doctor and helping determine the right antibiotics for what appears to be full-blown sepsis in Ms. Smith. You and the rest of the care delivery team know that this is a life-threatening infection. You and the doctor spend lots of time selecting the correct empiric regimen until the cultures and sensitivities come back. Two days later, Ms. Smith is hanging on by a tread in your intensive care unit. The sensitivities are back: the organism requires vancomycin and gentamycin, so you and the intensivist and infectious diseases doctor are collaborating and calculating the appropriate dosing regimen. After you begin the therapy, the patient seems to be responding well. Two days later, the patient is transferred to the med/surg unit where you are staffing that day. Discharge planners are actively working on how to appropriately transfer Ms. Smith home. Continuation of parenteral antibiotics will be needed after discharge, so you are consulted about how to do that safely. You and the internal medicine doctor agree that a percutaneous indwelling central catheter (PICC) line is needed to safely administer the antibiotics on an outpatient basis. You have met with the patient many times over her hospital stay and you and the internal medicine doctor agree that she is capable of being taught how to care for her PICC line prior to discharge. You and the rest of the care delivery team are actively working on placement of the PICC line and getting Ms. Smith ready for discharge.

Then the Director of Nursing (DNS) comes to talk to the care delivery team about Ms. Smith. She and the social worker inform you that Ms. Smith is intermittently homeless with a long history of drug abuse as evidenced by her frequent visits to the ED in the past few years. Many of the prior visits to the ED required her to be resuscitated from opiate overdoses. The DNS and social worker feel that sending Ms. Smith out on the street with a PICC line will be tantamount to signing her death warrant. They feel that Ms. Smith will abuse the easy access to her circulatory system to take more illicit drugs and quite possibly kill herself. The DNS informs the care delivery team they cannot discharge the patient with a PICC line. The admitting doctor (who happens to be the Chief of Staff) tells the DNS that the patient might likely die of infection if she can't continue her parenteral antibiotic regimen for the next 10 days (at least) and staying in the hospital is not acceptable for that length of time. You and the rest of the care delivery team observe the DNS and admitting doctor devolve into shouting argument about the appropriate care of Ms. Smith.

This is it. You feel you can help! You remember your training in ethical thinking from school. You know from this training that there is no right or wrong answer in ethical dilemmas, only carefully thought out answers to difficult clinical situations like this one. If you can step in and help mediate this (almost) unprofessional exchange between the patient's doctor and DNS, you would hit the "home run" you want: when you apply for the Director of Pharmacy job, both these individuals will remember your help delivering the best care possible for the patient and, at the same time, helping both leaders to work beyond their differences of opinion.

You realize this will be high-risk intervention. If you can't get the leaders to see that this is a simple ethical dilemma that just needs to be worked through, the opposite might happen, and you might be seen as an overly ambitious pharmacist making things even more complicated for this patient. You consider maybe letting them work it out on their own. Obviously, no one else on the care delivery team is sending any signals that they want to help these leaders solve the problem. They are all backing away from the growing ugly scene, or assuming a disengaged, head-down position working their cell phones.

Case Question/Instructions

What should you do next? So that this problem never occurs again, what would a long-term solution to this problem look like? Write your paper to solve this case, making sure you follow the directions provided by your instructor, and ensure that your paper provides all necessary information outlined in the assignment.

Subcategory: Professionalism

Chapter 4: Ethics

Case #59: Death with Dignity: Conscientious Objection

You are the manager of a local retail pharmacy that has been in business for years. You are in the office writing the next work schedule and your phone rings. It is a call from June, the distraught daughter of a long-time patient of your pharmacy. June is hysterical: "How could you?!" She is gasping for air as she accuses your pharmacy of being a cold, mean, and heartless business. You finally get a word in edgewise and ask her what happened. June collects her thoughts, takes a few deep breaths and begins her story.

"Last month, on the 5th, my mother came to your pharmacy—as she has done for the last 25 years—to get a prescription filled." This prescription was for pentobarbital capsules, which she was going to use to end her suffering from terminal cancer, a decision permitted under the state's Death with Dignity Act. Your pharmacist Mary refused to fill it! "Mary said it was against her religion to participate in an immoral activity such as filling Mom's prescription that would 'kill her.' How could Mary be so mean and cruel to my Mom in her moment of need?! Mary sent Mom to the pharmacy across town that she said would fill a prescription 'like this.' Mom was too sick to make the trip, so we had to schedule for Mom to go to that pharmacy the next time my brother was off work to take her. It took a week! Mary caused so much anxiety and stress in Mom that we had to take her to her doctor and get referred to a psychologist to help her get over it. Mom has struggled through Mary's outrageous decision and has since exercised her legal right to end her life and she has passed. But the stress and anxiety Mary created in my family in the final days of Mom's life are inexcusable. I ought to report your pharmacy to the Board! I should sue you!"

Case Question/Instructions

What should you do next? So that this problem never occurs again, what would a long-term solution to this problem look like? Write your paper to solve this case, making sure you follow the directions provided by your instructor, and ensure that your paper provides all necessary information outlined in the assignment.

In order to solve this case, the student(s) will need to imagine this case takes place in one of the states that have legalized death with dignity, and refer to those laws and rules that apply to the solution of this case.

Case #60: Principles of Autonomy vs Non-Maleficence

You are a staff pharmacist in a local retail pharmacy in a small coastal community with conservative values. You graduated from pharmacy school five years ago and have worked in this store since graduation. You know your patients and their families. One day, one of your customer's daughters, Destiny, comes in to pick up a prescription for her mother and she buys a few over-the-counter (OTC) drugs at the same time. As you are ringing her up, you see a package of condoms among the OTCs. You complete the transaction and ask her to join you in the private counseling booth in your pharmacy. You ask her if the condoms are for her. She says yes. You ask her if she has ever used them before. She says no. You don't remember exactly how old Destiny is, but she is probably 15 or 16 years old. You perform your usual and professional counseling to Destiny, the same as you would for anyone using condoms for the first time. Part of your counseling is to inform first time users of condoms about sexually transmitted diseases (STDs) and how condoms are highly effective at helping against the spread of STDs. You emphasize to Destiny that she should use condoms each and every time she has sex for the foreseeable future. You ask Destiny if you can open the box, so you can show her one of the condoms and how to use it. She says yes, and you demonstrate proper application by rolling the condom onto two of your fingers. It was an awkward conversation for Destiny, but she is grateful, and you did it with compassion and professionalism. It went well and Destiny leaves with her mother's meds and OTCs and her condoms.

The next day Destiny's mother storms into your pharmacy and pushes her way to the front of the line and shouts out your name! You come to the cash register and she slaps down the package of prescriptions, OTCs, and condoms you sold Destiny yesterday. "Did you sell these to my daughter?!" You ask the mother to join you in the private counseling booth. Destiny's mother proceeds to verbally attack you for selling condoms to her 14-year-old daughter. She tells you her values include sexual abstinence before marriage, and that your decision to sell condoms threatens those values and Destiny's reproductive health if she fails to use or improperly uses the condoms. She angrily demands that instead, you should have called her and informed her of Destiny's desire to buy condoms, so she could talk some sense into her! She is extremely distraught!

Case Question/Instructions

What should you say to Destiny's mother? So that this problem never occurs again, what would a long-term solution to this problem look like? Write your paper to solve this case, making sure you follow the directions provided by your instructor, and ensure that your paper provides all necessary information outlined in the assignment.

Case #61: Combative Mood of Peer

You work at a small independent pharmacy and have a coworker pharmacist who simply loses it at work and blows up at a patient for no reason that you can discern. The patient, who you have spoken to and calmed down, asks you for the name of the Pharmacist in Charge and says to you that she is going to file a complaint with the Store Manager and the Board of Pharmacy. You provide the patient with the name of the Pharmacist in Charge, as requested. This isn't the first time for your coworker. You fear he may get fired. The coworker has admitted to you in prior conversation that he suffers from a mood swing disorder, for which he is taking prescribed medication. Later, your coworker apologizes to you for having to deal with the issue and admits to you that he stopped taking his meds, but that now he sees that he needs to resume them. He tells you he will.

Case Question/Instructions

What should you do next? What would a long-term solution to this problem look like? Write your paper to solve this case, making sure you follow the directions provided by your instructor, and ensure that your paper provides all necessary information outlined in the assignment.

Case #62: Rashid and the Alleged Terrorist

You are a staff pharmacist in a retail pharmacy. The store owner, Rashid, is also a pharmacist and working alongside you today. You two get along and have a good personal relationship. Rashid openly talks about his childhood in a small village in Iraq. He is now a U.S. citizen, but remembers his homeland fondly. Over the years of working with Rashid, you have learned a great deal about the culture and traditions of his home village. You learned how he and his family left Iraq years ago and immigrated to the United States and became citizens. It is an inspiring story of how good, honest, hardworking poor immigrants adopted and embraced the United States as their homeland and succeeded. Over the years while sharing with you bits and pieces of his family's story, Rashid has explained a lot about his Muslim religion, not in any effort to convert you, but because you expressed curiosity and he obliged. Along the way, you learned the differences between Sunni and Shiite religious sects.

Today a new customer, Mr. Muhammed T'krit comes in with several prescriptions. Rashid greets the new customer with his normal and typical warmth. He reads the name of Mr. T'krit on the prescription and you observe him appear to be alarmed and become angry. Rashid calls out to Mr. T'krit using Arabic language. An energetic exchange between the two men begins. You don't understand Arabic, but you can tell by the volume and gestures that this is not a happy exchange. In fact, you can tell there is genuine anger between the two men. Rashid comes around the counter and stands toe to toe with Mr. T'krit, shouting angrily in Arabic. The shouting between the two men gets louder and you begin to wonder if it will come to a physical fight. You begin to come around the counter to try to calm things down when Rashid throws Mr. T'krit's prescriptions in his face and storms off. Mr. T'krit throws an obscene gesture back at Rashid, including what appears to be Arabic cursing, and storms out of the store.

You and the rest of the store employees are totally shocked! Nothing like this has ever happened before. After a few moments of stunned silence, you follow Rashid into his office. "What on Earth just happened out there, Rashid?"

Rashid is red in the face and actually trembling with anger. He takes a few deep breaths and asks you to sit down. Rashid tells you about a time in his home village in Iraq when an Iraqi soldier murdered his brother, in his own home, in front of his entire family. The soldier was looking for terrorists and thought Rashid's brother fit the description of a terrorist. The soldier's family name was T'krit and was a member of the other Muslim sect, different from Rashid's family. Rashid said he was trying to find out if Mr. T'krit was from his home village and when the answer was yes, Rashid accused Mr. T'krit's relative of the murder of his brother and the angry exchange grew from that. Still visibly angry, Rashid completed the discussion by saying he will never serve anyone from the other Muslim sect: "They are all killers and rapists!"

The next day you ask to talk to Rashid privately in his office. You point out that Mr. T'krit should not have been treated that way. Rashid angrily pushes back and tells you to not stick your nose in where it does not belong and orders you back to work.

Case Question/Instructions

What should you do next? So that this problem never occurs again, what would a long-term solution to this problem look like? Write your paper to solve this case, making sure you follow the directions provided by your instructor, and ensure that your paper provides all necessary information outlined in the assignment.

Case #63: Another Ethical Dilemma

You are Lynn, a pharmacist at a community pharmacy. You are working the evening shift when Mr. Benz calls in a refill for his temazepam. You see that there are two refills left on his prescription and you inform him that it will be ready tomorrow morning. About 20 minutes later, Mrs. Benz calls in and asks to speak with you. While whispering into the phone, Mrs. Benz pleads with you to not fill her husband's prescription, because Mr. Benz tried to commit suicide a couple of days ago and Mrs. Benz fears that he will use the temazepam to try again. You realize that the prescription is valid, and you feel an obligation to fill it, but Mrs. Benz's concern, if true, would be a problem. You assure Mrs. Benz that you will follow up about her concern appropriately. You do not say that you will or will not fill the prescription. Despite the vagueness of your reply, Mrs. Benz expresses relief and satisfaction with your commitment to follow up. After hanging up, you are perplexed. Should you fill the prescription? Should you call the police and have Mr. Benz arrested, committed to mental health facility? Should you refuse to fill the prescription? You forgot to ask Mrs. Benz if you could share her concern with her husband. You did not ask Mrs. Benz to do anything about her concern. You talk to your coworkers about the conversation you had with Mrs. Benz. The rest of the pharmacy staff are equally perplexed. Some say fill it, it is none of our business what Mr. Benz may or may not do with his temazepam. Others say don't fill it because we could be held liable for his death if he does commit suicide. Pharmacist John says that it is a valid prescription, and as such needs to be filled. He says that if we don't fill it or find someone who will, the Board of Pharmacy will fine us for obstructing the delivery of care! All agree that it would be appropriate to call the doctor who prescribed temazepam and talk this over. You call the doctor's office, but because it is evening, you can only leave a message.

You come to work the next morning and the first thing you do is check if the doctor for Mr. Benz's temazepam prescription called back. She has not. You call the doctor again and can only get as far as the doctor's nurse. The nurse says that the doctor is in the middle of an outpatient minor surgical procedure and is not available. You tell the story to the nurse and demand that the doctor call back as soon as she can, because Mr. Benz could be in at any moment. The nurse agrees to tell the doctor.

Ten minutes later, Mr. Benz comes into the store. The doctor has not called back. Mr. Benz is over at the beer and wine section buying a jug of wine. You know he is going to come to you next.

Case Question/Instructions

What should you say to Mr. Benz? So that this problem never occurs again, what would a long-term solution to this problem look like? Write your paper to solve this case, making sure you follow the directions provided by your instructor, and ensure that your paper provides all necessary information outlined in the assignment.

Case #64: Oxy Ethical Dilemma

Richard is married to Mary. They have been married for 20 years. They are both 50 years old. Mary has developed severe lower abdominal pain in the last week. Finally, she agrees to go to the emergency department (ED), at Richard's insistence. There she is given injectable opiate analgesics and taken for a CT scan. The diagnosis is confirmed: Mary is suffering from acute diverticulitis of the lower descending colon with complicating infected abscess. The ED doctor writes her a few prescriptions and advises Mary to see her Primary Care Provider right away for follow-up treatment. Richard collects his wife from the ED and takes her home. He notes that she is in an all-too-familiar euphoric state of mind from the opiate analgesics given in the ED. Mary is feeling wonderful and this is bad, very bad. Back in the day, both Mary and Richard abused heroin and, as is common, they both suffered through a serious decline in health and attending strain on family and friends. They developed a codependent relationship to help them get through the highs and lows of drug abuse. At about the same time, and after helping each other get through some life-threatening overdoses, they both decided to get clean and change their lives before they killed themselves. During their time together in rehab, their relationship changed, and they fell in love and eventually got married. Since then they have had a few relapses abusing drugs, but each spouse would help the other get cleaned up and back on track. Despite the struggles associated with being addicts, which they understand will last the rest of their lives, they have managed their disability pretty well and helped each other stay mostly clean since they were married. Richard is worried that Mary is reliving the euphoria of heroin on their way home from the ED.

Richard pulls into Best-way Pharmacy to get the prescriptions filled. There were three prescriptions: two are for antibiotics to combat the abscess in her colon, and one is oral oxycodone for pain control. You are Lisa, a pharmacist at Best-way Pharmacy. When you come to counsel Mary on the proper use of the drugs, Richard attends, with Mary's permission. Mary is still under the influence of the analgesics from the ED and could forget something you say. You talk them through the use of antibiotics and explain why it is important to finish all the prescribed doses. Then you go on to explain the use of oxycodone. As soon as Richard hears that the third prescription is for oxy, he stops you: "We don't want that prescription. Mary and I have a long history with abusing opiates and oxy will likely cause Mary to relapse. I'm already seeing many reminders of Mary's addictive behaviors from the dose given in the ED; we don't

Chapter 4: Ethics

want the oxy prescription." You explain that Mary's condition is quite painful and that she will need some powerful analgesics to get her through this episode of diverticular disease. Richard says that Mary will do fine with ibuprofen and acetaminophen. Richard goes on to say, "We have a right to refuse treatment we don't want, and we don't want the prescription for oxy." You turn to Mary, who seems to be humming a tune softly to herself in the corner of the consultation room. "Mary?" you ask. Mary lifts her head and smiles at you. You ask Mary if she agrees with what Richard has just said about refusing the oxy prescription. Mary says—actually kind of slurs— "But I need the oxy, my tummy hurts." Richard says that Mary is under the influence, she does not know what she is saying. "We refuse the oxy."

Case Question/Instructions

What should you do next? What would a long-term solution to this problem look like? Write your paper to solve this case, making sure you follow the directions provided by your instructor, and ensure that your paper provides all necessary information outlined in the assignment.

Case #65: Beneficence vs Veracity: Placebos

You are Manny, the owner/manager and staff pharmacist at a community pharmacy. You are the last independent pharmacy in the neighborhood; the other independent pharmacies sold out to the chain stores long ago. You have embraced the marketing strategy of personal service, honest business practice, and genuine connection with your patients and their families to survive the aggressive low-cost marketing strategies of the nearby chain pharmacies. Your business model has been largely successful. You have a steady clientele who cherish your open, honest, friendly neighborhood approach to pharmacy.

One of your patients, Mr. Tom Watson, suffers from lupus erythematosus, an autoimmune disorder that can affect a wide variety of organ systems. In Mr. Watson's case, a number of systems are being nearly constantly attacked by his own immune system. He suffers from classic symptoms of fatigue, joint and muscle pain, periodic painful skin rashes, sensitivity to light, headaches, and hair loss, just to name a few. You know this to be a chronic condition that Mr. Watson will be dealing with for the rest of his life. You have been very empathetic to Mr. Watson's condition and have spent lots of time explaining the drug regimens that his immunologist has prescribed over the years. Mr. Watson's doctor has changed up drug regimens to symptomatically treat Tom's condition and provide him with as much relief and rest as possible, particularly when Tom's condition flares up and he suffers new and different painful symptoms. It really is a difficult chronic disease and your heart goes out to Tom and his family. It is a poorly understood disease and many people think it is all in his head. Tom does not help himself either. He can overreact emotionally when new symptoms appear. Even some staff in your pharmacy appear to have little patience with Mr. Watson when he wants to vent about his symptoms. You, however, have always been totally engaged with Tom whenever he needed to talk. Not only because that is part of your business model, but additionally you genuinely care for Tom and his painful affliction.

Today, Tom's immunologist Dr. Stevens calls to talk to you about Tom. Tom has suffered a serious flare in his disease. Tom is in a great deal of pain and now suffers from symptoms of arthritis and Raynaud's syndrome. Dr. Stevens is concerned, because Tom is asking for and preoccupied with using opiate analgesics. Dr. Stevens does not want Tom to add addiction issues to his problem list. Dr. Stevens asks you to order some over-the-counter sleep/analgesic product with melatonin and acetaminophen, grind it up, make capsules and repackage it as a prescription and label it "Dr. Stevens' experimental remedy." Dr. Stevens is clearly going for a placebo effect by telling Mr. Watson that this new experimental remedy might be highly effective and that he should try it out. Dr. Stevens explains that Mr. Watson enthusiastically embraced this new experimental option. It is clear Dr. Stevens just wants to give Mr. Watson some rest and sleep to help him endure this latest lupus flare. Dr. Stevens indicates that he might change the formula of the remedy from time to time to add different and perhaps legend drugs to treat evolving symptoms and to overcome the inevitable treatment failure that will occur after prolonged use of the remedy. Dr. Stevens asks you up front if you will join him in this placebo-like therapy for Mr. Watson's condition. You are moved by Dr. Stevens' commitment to Mr. Watson's well-being and agree. As part of this plan, you agree not to share the ingredients of the remedy with Mr. Watson or his family so that this placebo-like plan has the best chance for success.

Eureka! It seems to be working. Mrs. Watson has come in for three refills of the remedy. Dr. Stevens only had to change the formula once, to add diphenhydramine for added sedative and antipruritic effects. The doses of all the ingredients are minimal and safe, and in all likelihood ineffective, but the placebo effect is powerful in Mr. Watson and it is working. Today Mrs. Watson brings in Mr. Watson in a wheelchair and both are in high spirits. Mr. Watson got out of bed today for the single reason of coming in to thank you, his pharmacist, for helping him get through this latest serious bout with his lupus. There are actual tears in his eyes when he feebly grasps your hand to express his thanks. His wife hugs you warmly and she expresses their thankfulness to you and your pharmacy for all that you are doing to help Tom. Several staff members overhear and watch the exchange and they too are tearing up with joy at what they are witnessing. Mr. Watson seems genuinely happy even though he is horribly afflicted with this latest flare up of lupus. Tom wants a refill of "the remedy" and asks you, "what is in this stuff anyway? It's a miracle!"

Case Question/Instructions

What should you say to Mr. Watson? What would a long-term solution to this problem look like? Write your paper to solve this case, making sure you follow the directions provided by your instructor, and ensure that your paper provides all necessary information outlined in the assignment.

Acknowledgements

No book is written in isolation. I wish to acknowledge my partners in this work, Michael Millard, Asst. Professor, Madeline Fry, Asst. Professor, and my wife Diane Arendt.

Without the contributions of these individuals, our work would have never made it as far as this book, and thus would never have reached our students. Indeed, this book would have failed to occur.

I am eternally grateful to all three individuals, whose insightful contributions to this text make it a valuable teaching tool for the rest of the world.

Steven J. Arendt

BIBLIOGRAPHY

Bibliography

By now you have confirmed what we stated earlier. This book does not attempt to teach leadership skills or specific techniques. Instead, this book sets up cases for students to apply what they have learned in other leadership courses, and allows experienced faculty to guide and coach students to reasonable, realistic solutions.

Having said that, it is important to provide students with a "leadership" library to enable them to perform the research needed to select the appropriate proven (i.e., published) leadership style(s) which supports their chosen solution.

Books

Bass, B. M., & Riggio, R. E. (2014). *Transformational leadership.* New York, NY: Routledge.

Blanchard, K. H., & Johnson, S. (2012). *The one minute manager.* London: HarperCollins.

Chisholm-Burns, M. A., Vaillancourt, A. M., & Shepherd, M. (2014). *Pharmacy management, leadership, marketing, and finance.* Burlington, MA: Jones & Bartlett Learning.

Clark, T., & White, S. J. (2015). *Wisdom from the pharmacy leadership trenches.* Bethesda, MD: American Society of Health-System Pharmacists.

Collins, J. (2001). *Good to great: Why some companies make the leap ... and others don't.* London: Random House.

Covey, S. R. (2016). *The 7 habits of highly effective people.* Selangor: PTS Publishing House.

DeCoske, M., Tryon, J., & White, S. J. (2014). *Pharmacy leadership field guide cases and advice for everyday situations.* Bethesda, MD: American Society of Health-System Pharmacists.

Dye, C. F., & Garman, A. N. (2015). *Exceptional leadership: 16 critical competencies for healthcare executives.* Chicago, IL: Health Administration Press.

Goleman, D., Mckee, A., & Boyatzis, R. (2003). *Primal leadership: Realizing the power of emotional intelligence.* Seoul: Chung Rim Publishing.

Harter, J., & Buckingham, M. (2016). *First, break all the rules: What the world's greatest managers do differently.* New York, NY: Gallup Press.

Heifetz, R. A., Grashow, A., & Linsky, M. (2009). *The practice of adaptive leadership: Tools and tactics for changing your organization and the world.* Boston, MA: Harvard Business Press.

Hennessy, J. E. (1992). *Competitive servant leadership: A quality concept.* Indianapolis, IN: Robert K. Greenleaf Center

Kotter, J. P. (2012). *Leading change.* Boston, MA: Harvard Business Review Press.
Kouzes, J. M., & Posner, B. Z. (2011). *The five practices of exemplary leadership: Healthcare—general.* Somerset: Wiley.

Kouzes, J. M., & Posner, B. Z. (2017). *The leadership challenge: How to make extraordinary things happen in organizations.* Hoboken, NJ: Wiley.

Ledlow, G. R., & Stephens, J. H. (2018). *Leadership for health professionals: Theory, skills, and applications.* Burlington, MA: Jones & Bartlett Learning.

Lencioni, P. (2007). *The five dysfunctions of a team: Team assessment*. San Francisco: Pfeiffer.

Maxwell, J. C. (n.d.). *The 21 irrefutable laws of leadership: Follow them and people will follow you*. Nashville, TN: Thomas Nelson.

McChesney, C., Covey, S., & Huling, J. (2016). *The 4 disciplines of execution: Achieving your wildly important goals*. New York, NY: Free Press.

Patterson, K., Grenny, J., McMillan, R., & Switzler, A. (2012). *Crucial conversations: Tools for talking when stakes are high*. Singapore: McGraw-Hill Education.

Rath, T., & Conchie, B. (2009). *Strengths based leadership: Great leaders, teams, and why people follow*. New York, NY: Gallup Press.

Sinek, S. (2013). *Start with why: How great leaders inspire everyone to take action*. London: Portfolio/Penguin.

Zgarrick, D. P., Moczygemba, L. R., Alston, G. L., & Desselle, S. P. (2016). *Pharmacy management: Essentials for all practice settings*. New York, NY: McGraw-Hill Education.

Articles

Kotter, J. P. (1990). What leaders really do. *Harvard Business Review, 68*(3), 103–111.

White, S. J. (2009). Your professional practice vision. *American Journal of Health-System Pharmacy, 66(16), 1432–1435*.

Zilz, D. A., Woodward, B. W., Thielke, T. S., Shane, R. R., & Scott, B. (2004). Leadership skills for a high-performance pharmacy practice. *American Journal of Health-System Pharmacy, 61*(23), 2562–2574.

www.ingramcontent.com/pod-product-compliance
Lightning Source LLC
Chambersburg PA
CBHW081728100526
44591CB00016B/2545